"If it hadn't been for his innate sense of humor—brilliantly demonstrated in this memoir of his Mayo residency—and a sense of perspective derived from that experience, he might have failed. He didn't and here he honors those who helped him along the way and those whom he helped. If Collins's scalpel is as sharp as his pen, his patients are in capable hands indeed."

—*Booklist*

"A fast-paced memoir of the fear, heartbreak, humor, and triumph."

—*Notre Dame Magazine*

"I adore this book. It's so polished and hilarious. It brought back all the stomach-churning anxieties of my own residency so vividly that I felt exhausted reading it. Dr. Collins has my highest admiration. I give this book a 10+!"

—Tess Gerritsen, *New York Times* bestselling author of *The Surgeon*

"One of the best, funniest medical memoirs I have ever read. *Hot Lights, Cold Steel* is at once darkly humorous and truly compassionate. Not since *The House of God* has there been such a ferociously funny look at the world of hospital medicine."

—Michael Palmer, *New York Times* bestselling author of *Fatal* and *The Patient*

"Like the very best episode of *ER*, Collins's memoir races from one trauma to the next, keeping this reader spellbound all the way. Collins's life as a surgical resident is heartbreaking one minute and triumphant the next. You'll laugh and cry and cheer along with him as his epic journey to become a doctor races toward its gripping conclusion. I love this book and won't soon forget it."

—Augusten Burroughs, *New York Times* bestselling author of *Dry* and *Magical Thinking*

www.stmartins.com

Library of Congress Cataloging-in-Publication Data

Collins, Michael J., M.D.
    Hot lights, cold steel : life, death and sleepless nights in a surgeon's first years / Michael J. Collins.
        p. cm.
    ISBN 0-312-33778-7 (hc)
    ISBN 0-312-35269-7 (pbk)
    EAN 978-0-312-35269-1
    1. Collins, Michael, J., M.D. 2. Orthopedists—United States—Biography. 3. Surgeons—United States—Biography. I. Title.

RD728.C64A3 2005
617.4'7'092—dc22
[B]
                                                                    2004051247

First St. Martin's Griffin Edition: February 2006

10  9  8  7  6  5  4  3  2  1

# Hot Lights, Cold Steel

*Life, Death and Sleepless Nights
in a Surgeon's First Years*

Michael J. Collins, M.D.

*David Graulich
Fair Oaks, CA
August 9, 2021*

ST. MARTIN'S GRIFFIN ⚑ NEW YORK

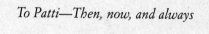

*To Patti—Then, now, and always*

We start here, and we go there. But it's not that simple, is it? Our paths may be circuitous or direct. We may gaze excitedly ahead, or cast our eyes regretfully behind. Until we reach our destination it exists only in our own minds. It is what we have imagined it to be. And yet we tend to neglect the journey, which is real, in favor of the destination, which is not.

For too long I neglected this journey. It was an obstacle to be overcome, an ordeal to be endured; for I had never chosen the journey, I had chosen the destination. But now that the journey has ended, I have discovered that *here* isn't so important after all. I find myself looking back with particular fondness for how I got here.

St. Mary's Hospital Emergency Room
The Mayo Clinic, Rochester, Minnesota
June, Year Four

*The ER doors crashed open and the paramedics powered through. I trotted alongside them as they wheeled the patient to Trauma One.*

*"Fourteen-year-old kid, run over by a tractor," the paramedic said. "He was conscious when we got there, BP a hundred over sixty. His right leg's a mess—open fracture, dirt everywhere."*

*"What's his name?" I asked.*

*"Johannson. Kenny Johannson."*

*"Hang in there, Kenny," I whispered to the unconscious boy.*

*I lifted the sheet covering the lower half of his body, and immediately the thick, fetid stink of manure mushroomed up at me. His leg was twisted obscenely to the side. The jagged end of the tibia stuck through a rent in his dirty blue jeans. A spreading pool of blood soaked the sheet underneath him.*

*As we lifted the boy onto the table in Trauma One, his eyes flickered open. He began to whimper softly as he searched for someone he knew. I put my hand on the side of his head and rubbed his hair gently. "Kenny, you're in the emergency room at St. Mary's," I told him. "Your mom and dad are here, too. They're in the other room."*

*He rolled his head and moaned. "My leg. Oh, God, my leg! It hurts so bad."*

"I know it does, Kenny, and we are going to help you."

"BP seventy-eight over forty," a nurse called out. "Pulse one-sixty."

I probed Kenny's wound. Under the severed end of the peroneus longus there was a bloody chunk of manure wedged against the bone. I picked it up with a forceps and dropped it on the floor. When I found what was left of the anterior tibial artery I clipped it with a hemostat. His bleeding, except for a slow ooze, ceased.

In the next several minutes we did a cut-down, put in a subclavian line, and pumped him full of blood and fluid. Within half an hour we had his pressure up to one-ten over sixty. I told the charge nurse to get an OR ready. As she picked up the phone, she said the boy's parents wanted to talk to me.

Mr. and Mrs. Johannson were huddled together on a couch in the far corner of the waiting room. They sprang to their feet as I entered the room. Mrs. Johannson wrapped both hands around her husband's left arm and leaned against him. She kept staring at the bloodstains on my scrub pants.

I introduced myself and then told them that although Kenny had lost a lot of blood, his vital signs had improved and he seemed stable. "We are just about to take him to the operating room," I said.

Before I could say more, the door to the waiting room burst open and a young man rushed in. "Dad!" he said. "I found it."

"This is my son Eric," Mr. Johannson said. "He went back to the farm to look for the missing piece of Kenny's leg."

Eric reached into the pocket of his jacket. He handed me a clean white handkerchief in which he had wrapped a dirty, three-inch section of tibia. I doubted we could use it, but I wanted the boy to feel he had done something worthwhile. "Thanks, Eric," I said. "This could be a big help."

"Will you be able to save Kenny's leg?" Mr. Johannson asked.

At that moment I was more worried about saving Kenny's life. The boy was in shock and had almost bled to death. I longed to reassure his parents, but I had learned not to make promises. "Mr. Johannson," I said, "we're going to do everything we can."

"Please, Doc. Please."

I nodded, shook his hand, squeezed Mrs. Johannson's shoulder, and sprinted up to the OR.

They had taken Kenny to OR Ten, the largest of the operating rooms. In contrast to the ER, where everyone had been barking orders, shouting for equipment, and rushing back and forth, the operating room was quiet, almost hushed. Voices were muffled. There was a greater sense of control here. We were surgeons. This was our turf.

Against the far wall the laminar-flow machine hummed faintly. The cardiac monitor issued its staccato, reassuring beeps. Two anesthesiologists were wedged shoulder to shoulder at the head of the table. They had just finished the intubation. The scrub nurse stood at the back table carefully arranging her instruments. Two circulating nurses shuttled back and forth with instrument trays from the sterilizer. In the corner, a radiology tech waited patiently next to her portable X-ray machine.

I handed the piece of tibia to the circulating nurse and asked her to sterilize it. Then I scrubbed my hands and joined the five other residents from various surgical specialties who were clustered around the shattered leg. The extent of the boy's injuries was now apparent. Large sections of muscle, skin, and bone were missing. Parts of nerves and arteries had been torn away. Dirt, manure, and fertilizer contaminated everything.

First one, then another of the residents poked at the wound, winced or shook his head, then stepped back. No one was sure what to do. Should we try to save this leg, or should we amputate it?

They all looked at me. I was the chief resident in Orthopedic Surgery. I was the one who had to decide.

I stood in the center of the operating room with the bright lights trained on the bloody mess that was Kenny's leg. I tried to put everything else out of my mind. It didn't matter how much sleep I got the night before. It didn't matter what else I had planned for the rest of the day. This poor kid, barely alive, was lying unconscious on an operating table with some stranger about to decide whether to cut off his leg.

I hemmed and hawed for a few minutes. The natural impulse, of course, is to save the leg. If there is a chance in a million, take it. The kid was only fourteen years old. What did we have to lose by trying? If it didn't work *we could always amputate the leg later. Didn't we owe him at least that much?*

*I wasn't sure. Kenny's leg was so badly damaged that an attempt to save his leg could cost him his life.*

*But what about Kenny? What would he want? If we woke him up and said, "Kenny, your leg is severely injured. Should we cut it off or try to save it?" Did anyone think he would say, "Cut it off"?*

*For Christ's sake, he was only fourteen years old.*

*The room was quiet save for the sigh of the ventilator and the steady beep of the cardiac monitor. From behind the drape at the head of the table, the anesthesiologists looked at me questioningly. The other residents stood silent, some looking at the ground, some staring at the gaping wound in front of us. No one moved. No one spoke. They all waited.*

# YEAR ONE

# CHAPTER ONE

*The Mayo Clinic, Rochester, Minnesota*
*July, Four Years Earlier*

On a sweltering Friday afternoon, the day before we were to officially begin our residency, we gathered in a small classroom on the fourteenth floor of the Mayo Building for our orientation meeting. Crammed into this room were fifteen incredibly bright first-year orthopedic surgery residents—and me, a twenty-nine-year-old ex-cabdriver and ex-construction worker long on dreams but short on credentials.

We were introduced one by one. *Phi Beta* this, *Alpha Omega* that. The Mayo Clinic was the most prestigious medical center in the world, and I began to wonder what I was doing there. I was the redheaded stepchild, the dullest scalpel in the drawer.

All the other residents had done several rotations in orthopedics when they were in medical school. Most of them had spent their nights writing papers or doing orthopedic research. When I was in medical school I had spent my nights working on a truck dock. I had done no research, had written no papers, and had done only one rotation in ortho. I had no exposure to the world of adult reconstructive surgery that was such a big part of orthopedics at the Mayo Clinic.

After the introductions, a towering man with thick lips and wavy gray hair lumbered up to the podium. He introduced himself as Dr. John

Harding, the chairman of the department. He welcomed us and then gave a brief history of orthopedic surgery at Mayo, going all the way back to Drs. Will and Charlie Mayo, who had founded the Clinic in the 1890s. He said we were lucky to be starting in orthopedics now. "Twenty years ago there were no joint replacements. There was no arthroscopy. The things we can do for our patients now could scarcely have been imagined back when I started in orthopedics."

When Dr. Harding finished, a short, wrinkle-faced man with thick glasses approached the microphone. He waited until the room was quiet before he introduced himself. "I am Dr. Benjamin Burke," he said, "the director of the residency program." After a few words of welcome, he reminded us of the sacredness of our profession, and told us we had a long, but gratifying, road ahead of us. "You will spend four years here," he said. "Two years as a junior resident, and two as a senior resident. If you work hard enough, if you're skilled enough, we might consider you for chief resident in your final year." He concluded by saying, "This is the Mayo Clinic. Our patients expect a lot from us, and we are going to expect a lot from you."

Finally, Viola Hopkins, Dr. Burke's secretary, passed out our first-quarter assignments.

"There are two Mayo Clinic hospitals," Vi said. "You will spend time at both hospitals, but for the first quarter, twelve of you have been assigned to St. Mary's Hospital. The remaining four will be at Rochester Methodist Hospital." She said she looked forward to meeting each of us personally, and wished us a "happy and blessed four years here at Mayo."

I tore open my packet. There were four names under the heading Rochester Methodist Hospital:

> Chapin, William T.
> Collins, Michael J.
> Manning, John F.
> Wales, Frank

As we filed out of the classroom someone tapped me on the shoulder.

"Mike Collins?"

"Yeah," I said, turning around.

A stocky, freckle-faced man with an unruly mass of red hair held out his hand. "Bill Chapin," he said. "I guess we're going to be inmates together."

As we shook hands Bill said, "Have you met these two characters yet?" He gestured behind him.

A friendly-looking guy with a bushy brown mustache and a string tie smiled and took my hand in both of his. "Wales," he said. "Frank Wales. It's a gol-dern pleasure to meet you." Frank, as I was to learn, was a Wyoming farmboy with a big smile and a bigger heart. I never could figure out how much of his country-boy shtick was put on and how much was genuine.

"And I'm Jack Manning," said a tall, athletic-looking man with round glasses and a receding hairline. I shook hands with Jack, too, who then asked me where I was from.

"Chicago," I said. "The West Side. How about you?"

"Corn country. Des Moines, Iowa."

I turned back to Frank Wales. "Frank, where are you from?"

"I'm from God's country—"

"You're from Chicago, too?"

"Chicago? Why, son, I'm from Wyoming, Wind River Country. Home of elk and bison and wild mustang and mountain peaks stretching as far and as high as the eye can see. I don't reckon you have anything like that in Chicago."

I said no, but we had some pretty big rats and cockroaches.

After the others left I went back to the residents' lounge and looked through the rest of my packet. I knew that each staff (or "attending") surgeon at Mayo had his own list of patients: his service. A senior resident and a junior resident were assigned to each surgeon. I was dismayed to learn I would be the junior resident with Dr. Harding.

Oh, great, I thought. Just what I need, to have the chairman of the department find out what a dope he has hired. I imagined him grilling me the next day.

"How much research have you done, Dr. Collins?"

"Research? Well, I haven't actually—"

"What about papers, then? Have you written anything?"

"Papers? Have I written papers? Well, not exactly. That is, ahem, not a lot. Well, maybe a little here and there, but nothing all that important. Of course I've been meaning to write them. Lots of them, in fact. I have some ideas, but I've been—" At that point I would let him know that my people would be getting back to his people on this. Soon.

Fortunately, Dr. Harding, or Big John, as the residents called him, took very little notice of me the next morning. After a perfunctory handshake, he directed his attention to the senior resident, Art Hestry. Art led us up to the ortho floor to make rounds on our patients. At Mayo, rounds are made twice a day. The attending surgeon accompanies his residents on rounds every morning except Sunday. The residents make rounds by themselves every afternoon plus Sunday morning.

As we stood outside the first patient's room, Art gave Dr. Harding a brief summary: "TKA, day 2. Hemovac out. Up today. Doing well." This apparently meant something to Dr. Harding, who nodded and strode into the room. I shuffled after them wondering what the hell a TKA was.

By staying in the background and keeping my mouth shut, I managed to make it through rounds without making my ignorance too obvious. But I was a sober, frightened young man when we finished rounds that morning. I had a lot of catching up to do.

To make matters worse, there was the matter of the Saturday Morning Conference. Dr. Burke had warned us that all residents were required to attend this conference. I made my way to the hospital auditorium, where the conference was just beginning. One of the senior residents was presenting cases. I was in awe of his self-assurance and his command of orthopedic jargon.

"This is a fifty-two-year-old farmer, status-post right medial meniscectomy thirty years ago. He presents with a ten-year history of progressive DJD of the medial compartment. Dr. Coventry did a closing-wedge UTO last Wednesday."

I sat there in a daze, certain I was the most ignorant orthopedic resident in the history of the Mayo Clinic. I feverishly scribbled notes to myself: "UTO—??" and "Check X-rays on John Svendsen."

I was familiar with this type of conference from medical school. Cases are presented, then some unfortunate junior resident is asked a series of complex questions that he stammers through and always gets wrong. The senior resident or attending then gives the correct answer. Embarrassing the junior resident is considered a good thing. It is supposed to encourage him to study harder.

But I was another story. Although I had been an excellent student in medical school, I had very little exposure to orthopedics. After hearing the impressive qualifications of my fellow residents, I began to think my problems went beyond mere inexperience. Compared to the others, I felt orthopedically anencephalic. I felt brain dead with the plug pulled. I felt so ignorant that had anyone called on me even my questioner would have been embarrassed. The entire department would shudder if they discovered this moron was one of them.

At one point, Jack Manning, who was sitting behind me, leaned forward and asked how many UTOs I had scrubbed on. I pretended not to hear him. He might as well have asked how many UFOs I had flown on. At least I knew what a UFO was.

I don't think it is possible for a person to shrink down any farther in his seat than I did that morning. By the end of the conference my head was below the seat back. As we were leaving Jack said it looked like I was melting. But at least I hadn't been called on. My secret was safe for another week.

Even though the conference was over, I slunk out of the auditorium with my head down, still afraid someone might call me back and ask me under what circumstances would a hemi-arthroplasty be preferable to a total shoulder replacement? I would have thrown myself on the floor and asked them to shoot me and put me out of my misery.

And misery it was. In less than twenty-four hours I had gone from the euphoria of beginning my career as an orthopedic resident at the Mayo Clinic to the feeling I was a counterfeit, an impostor who had infiltrated this society of brilliant surgeons. Once my ignorance was discovered I would be told to report immediately to the director of the residency program. I would be ushered into a dimly lit room lined with cherrywood bookshelves crammed with faded, leather-bound medical treatises from the 1700s. A somber-looking Dr. Burke would emerge from the shadows and tell me a mistake had been made, a terrible mistake. He would then hand me an ornately carved wooden box.

"Go ahead," he would say. "Open it."

I would lift the lid and find a twelve-inch, pearl-handled dagger, its blade glinting wickedly, resting on a tiny satin pillow.

For the good of the residency program, for the good of the Mayo Clinic, for the good of every orthopedic surgeon who had ever picked up a scalpel, I would be urged to "do the right thing." Dr. Burke couldn't promise anything, of course, but if I "played ball," if I was "a team player," there was a chance my body would be given "first table" in the cadaver lab.

I went back to the doctors' lounge and began copying the list of patients on Dr. Harding's service. I planned to go back and review the chart on every patient. I had just finished copying the list when Art Hestry came in.

"Mike," he said, clapping me on the back. "I'm going up to the Twin Cities for the weekend. I need you to cover for me. I'll do rounds this afternoon before I leave, but you'll have to make rounds tomorrow."

He must have seen the look of horror on my face. "Don't worry. If you have any problems, just call one of the senior residents, they'll help you."

He laughed, handed me his beeper, said, "*Heck* of a deal!" and sailed out the door.

I stood there for several seconds, staring at this horrible thing, this beeper that rested in my still-outstretched hand. Gingerly, as if I were holding a vial of nitroglycerine, I clipped it to my belt. I was terrified that at any moment it might go off and a frantic nurse would scream, "Doctor, come quickly! Mr. Arnold's TQF is trans-debilitating on his acute dorsi! His TKA is UTO'd! For God's sake, hurry!"

I spent the rest of the day reviewing charts, slowly gleaning bits of information, jotting down on my ever-present index cards things like "TKA = Total Knee Arthroplasty," "ORIF = Open Reduction Internal Fixation," "UTO = Upper Tibial Osteotomy." Some things, however, defied my best efforts to decipher them. "Patient is TTWB," I read. Too tired with bending? Three times without bleeding? Terribly thirsty without beer? How in the hell did I know? Of course I could have asked the nurses, but they would have thrown me out the door for practicing medicine without a brain.

At six o'clock I pulled into the driveway of our small frame house on the outskirts of Rochester. My wife, Patti, met me at the back door. Patti and I were both Chicago kids, West Side Irish, born at St. Ann's Hospital at Lavergne and Thomas. Over her parents' strenuous objections, Patti had married me in the summer before my junior year in medical school.

"So," she said, throwing her arms around my neck, "how was your first day as an orthopedic surgeon?"

I cringed. I realized that only by the farthest stretch of the imagination could I be considered an orthopedic surgeon. There were medical students who knew more orthopedics than I did. I kissed Patti and mumbled that my first day was "okay."

"Then why the sad face? What did you do—operate on the wrong leg or something?"

"Aw, I don't know, hon. I feel so dumb, so out of it. I don't know the first thing about orthopedics."

Patti rubbed the back of her hand against my cheek. "That's why they have residencies."

One of the third-year ortho residents, John Stevenson, was giving a party that night. He had been thoughtful enough to invite the first-year guys. Patti and I left our twelve-month-old daughter, Eileen, with a babysitter. At eight o'clock we rang the doorbell of the Stevensons' apartment.

"Come on in," said the guy who answered the door. "John's in the kitchen."

The place was packed. It took me five minutes to find John. I handed him a six-pack of Olympia. He thanked me but said he hoped he wouldn't need it. There was a keg in the kitchen.

Patti and I stumbled around, listening to snippets of conversation about things called IM rods and Putti-Platts and ACLs. God, how I longed to find someone who could talk about the Vikings or the North Stars. At least I could speak the language.

We passed one of the residents on the hand service. He was talking about an operation they had done on a woman who had cut off her thumb in a lawn-mower accident. He said they removed her big toe and sewed it on her hand. I looked around. No one was laughing. The guy was serious.

In the kitchen I finally found Bill, Frank, and Jack. They lifted their glasses in greeting and we introduced our wives.

Alice Chapin, a strikingly beautiful woman, was a redhead, like Bill. I learned later that she had given up a promising career in public relations to move to Rochester. She had just gotten a job at the Rochester Public Library.

Jack Manning's wife, Sue, had warm hazel eyes and short brown hair. She was even more athletic looking than her husband. They had married right out of college. Jack told us they were expecting their first child in March.

"March?" Bill said, counting the months on his fingers. "When did Sue get pregnant, last night?"

The biggest surprise was Linda Wales, Frank's wife. Linda was an architect. In her crisp blouse and tight skirt, she was as sophisticated and polished as Frank was simple and rough-hewn. They had married when Frank was in medical school and Linda was getting her graduate degree.

John Stevenson, passing by, noticed I was drinking a Coke.

"Don't you want a beer, Mike?"

"Nah. I'm on call."

"On your first night? Junior residents only take call in-house. You can't be on call."

"Art Hestry went up to the Cities for the weekend. He gave me his beeper and left me on call for our service."

"He *what*?" John then called over several other senior residents. He introduced me, then told them Art had left me with the beeper for the weekend.

They all laughed. "Typical Art," they said. "Heck of a deal!"

A minute later, just as I found the pretzels, my beeper went off. I was so startled I almost dropped the bowl. The operator instructed me to call the ortho floor at Methodist. Oh, God, I thought, this is it. Someone's going to tell me I have to rush over to Methodist Hospital and perform some emergency operation I've never even heard of.

Heart pounding, I held my Coke over my head and squeezed through the crush of people in John's kitchen. I found a telephone in the bedroom, closed the door, and dialed the number.

"Dr. Collins," I said to the nurse who answered.

"Dr. Collins?" came the puzzled reply. "We were looking for Dr. Hestry."

"I'm covering for him."

"You are?" she said. "And this is Dr. Collins? I don't think I know you."

"Well, I just started today. I'm Dr. Harding's junior resident."

"Oh. Okay," she said reasonably, and then went on very businesslike. "I'm Ann Cheevers, the nurse taking care of Mrs. Wiltshire. Can we get her up?"

I frantically searched my memory. Mrs. Wiltshire. Mrs. Wiltshire. I vaguely remembered the name. I stalled and finally mumbled, "Mrs. Wiltshire . . . ?"

"Yes, Mrs. Wiltshire, in 7214. She had a TKA three days ago."

TKA, I thought in a panic. Oh, yeah, total knee arthroplasty.

Well, at least I knew what it was, but could we get her up? I hadn't a clue. I didn't know if "we" always got people up on the third day or if we never did. Mrs. Wiltshire was probably the wife of the president of Switzerland or something. What if I did the wrong thing? I could see the headlines of the Rochester *Post-Bulletin* the next day:

**IDIOT JUNIOR RESIDENT MISTAKENLY LETS
WIFE OF SWISS PRESIDENT WALK ON THIRD DAY. LEG FALLS OFF.**

I'd be finished. My career at Mayo would have lasted one day—although I would have to stay in Rochester for years while the malpractice trial dragged on. "Tell the ladies and gentlemen of the jury one more time, *Doctor,* how you crippled this poor mother of ten who had just won the Nobel Peace Prize."

I had been silent for quite a while when the nurse finally said, "Hello? Are you still there?"

"Uh, yeah. I'm still here."

"Well, can we get her up or not?"

There was no point in thinking it over. There was no way I could rationally discover an answer. Instead, I did the smartest thing I could have done: I threw myself on the mercy of the nurse.

"Look, Ann," I said, "I'm new and I honestly don't know. What do you usually do?"

This was her chance. She probably had been humiliated more than once by some egotistical resident. Now was her chance to get some payback.

I waited. She was silent for a moment and then must have taken pity on me. She let the opportunity to humiliate me pass. It wasn't the first time a nurse had helped me and it wouldn't be the last.

"We usually let them up. She's been doing fine. I think Dr. Hestry just forgot to write the order."

"Oh. Okay. Then it's fine. You can get her up."

"Thank you, Doctor."

I let out a long breath. "I owe you one, Ann."

"That's all right," she said with a laugh. "So where's Art?"

I wasn't sure if "covering" for Art meant lying for him, too. "Art? Oh. Well, Art is, uh . . ."

"Yes?"

"He . . . Well, he can't come to the phone right now."

"Yes, of course. I suppose he's desperately ill. Tell him I hope he feels better soon."

"I will."

"Tell him a couple aspirin and an ice pack on the forehead tomorrow morning might help."

"Well, I'm sure Art would never—"

"Good night, Doctor."

I hung up the phone and breathed a sigh of relief. I had passed my first test—barely. I went out to the living room and thanked John for inviting me. Then Patti and I headed home. I wanted to get a good night's sleep. The next morning I had to make rounds on every one of Dr. Harding's patients—by myself.

# CHAPTER TWO

*The next day*

The moment of truth had arrived. Art was out of town, Dr. Harding was sleeping, and rounds needed to be made. That left me, the greenest rookie imaginable, in charge.

We had fifteen patients on our service. Most of them had hip or knee replacements—operations I had never even seen. I just wanted to get through the morning without making some terrible mistake. I decided to make rounds so early that the patients would be too sleepy to ask me any questions. I was terrified one of them might ask me something like "Doctor, when can I resume dancing (or driving, or sex) after my hip (or knee, or shoulder) replacement?"

I couldn't just say, "Beats the hell out of me." I would have to come up with an answer. "Well, Mr. Spencer, resumption of activity following total hip replacement depends on a myriad of important factors." I would stroke my chin and pace slowly back and forth at the foot of his bed. "One must consider the integrity of the neuroprocesses, and the coefficient of friction of the metallic implant—not to mention the specific gravity of the synovial fluid. These are very complex issues. I will ask Dr. Harding to discuss this with you on Monday morning."

It was 4:57 A.M. when I pulled into the parking lot at the west end of

Methodist Hospital. As I walked in the back door, the security guard at the desk looked up from his magazine. "Emergency, huh, Doc?"

"Ah . . ." It was easier simply to agree. "Yeah, emergency," I said—which was true. If I didn't make it through rounds that morning I would be unemployed, and for me that would be a major emergency.

I went into the doctors' lounge and was panicked to find there were no computer lists. I found out later they weren't printed until 6:30 each morning. I had the list from the day before, but what if some French diplomat or Arabian sheik had been admitted during the night? What if he called Dr. Harding at the symphony or the golf course later that day demanding to know why no one had shown up to treat the green fungus on his femur?

My footsteps echoed down the dark halls as I made my way to the ortho floor. One of the nurses saw me pulling a chart from the rack.

"Is anything wrong, Doctor?"

"No. I'm just making rounds."

"Making rounds—at ten after five?"

"I wanted to get an early start."

She shook her head and went back to her charting.


I stood outside the first patient's room for several minutes, carefully reviewing the chart, checking outputs, vital signs, progress notes, and therapy records. Then I let out a slow breath and went in.

"Mr. Radcliff?"

No response.

I tried again, a little louder. "Mr. Radcliff?"

Finally, I reached over and shook his forearm. "Mr. Radcliff!"

"Huh?"

"Hi, Mr. Radcliff. It's Dr. Collins."

"Who?"

"Dr. Collins, remember? I'm one of the residents with Dr. Harding."

"Oh, yeah. Dr. Connolly. Is something wrong?"

"No, sir. I'm just here to check on you. Mind if I take a look at your incision?"

And so it went, patient after sleepy patient. I had a list of things Dr. Harding wanted done. ("Get her drain out tomorrow." "Change his dressing." "Put him in a cast.") Things went pretty well until I got to Lavinia Allenbaum's room. Mrs. Allenbaum was an eighty-two-year-old woman from a nursing home in Byron. She had fallen in the bathtub and fractured her hip. Dr. Harding had fixed it four days earlier.

She was sitting up in bed, picking at her blanket, as I entered the room.

"Good morning, Mrs. Allenbaum. I'm—"

"You're a no-good, lying son of a bitch. That's what you are."

I jerked to a halt. I felt like I had been slugged in the stomach. "Mrs. Allenbaum, if I have done anything to—"

"You've done everything. You and the rest of them. This is the worst hotel in Milwaukee. I'm never coming back to this place again."

The worst hotel in Milwaukee? Well, that explained things. Maybe I shouldn't take it personally when she said I was a lying son of a bitch.

I smiled reassuringly and went over to check her incision. I carefully lifted the edge of her hospital gown, and pulled back the dressing. The incision was healing nicely.

Mrs. Allenbaum slapped my hand. "What do you think you're doing? Why you little—"

"Sorry, Mrs. Allenbaum. I just needed to check your incision."

"Pervert! *Pervert!*" She was swinging her left hand at me, making the IV pole totter precariously.

"Mrs. Allenbaum, please. I'm one of your doctors."

"You're a filthy pervert. That's what you are!"

I backed away, waving my hands at her. She was shouting so loud that everyone on the floor must have heard that Mrs. Allenbaum's doctor was a filthy pervert. "Shhh, Mrs. Allenbaum. Shhh! You don't have to—" I backed right into a nurse who had come to investigate the commotion.

"Well, you got old Livy riled up now," the nurse said.

I held up my hands. "All I did was check her incision." I prayed the nurse hadn't already called the Vice Squad and the SWAT team to arrest the sicko who was molesting the old lady in 7203. Even now, 250-pound guys with huge biceps and black stockings pulled over their faces might be rappelling down the walls of the hospital, waiting to point machine guns at me and shout, "Freeze, turkey!" I would end my second day at the Mayo Clinic in the Sex Offenders Unit of the Olmsted County Jail.

"Relax," the nurse said. "Livy's a little confused this morning. An hour ago she pulled out her IV and then tried to bite me when I restarted it."

Mrs. Allenbaum, clutching her gown to her chest, continued to glare at me as I backed out of the room. There were only two more patients left to see. Was I imagining things or were they looking at me funny?

By 7:30 I was back in the doctors' lounge checking Dr. Harding's new list. Thankfully, no French diplomats or Arabian sheiks had been admitted during the night. John Stevenson, looking a little worse for wear, was tearing out his patient list from the printer. I thanked him for the party the night before and told him I had a good time.

"Are you making rounds today?" he asked.

"Just finished."

"Just finished? When did you start, six A.M.?"

"No, five."

"Are you nuts? Nobody makes rounds at five o'clock on Sunday."

When I told John why I had rounded so early, he nodded in understanding.

"Listen," he said, "you're gonna do fine. Stop worrying. First of all, orthopods aren't like fleas. Everyone isn't out to pimp you every minute of every day."

"Flea" is a pejorative term for an internist. Surgeons claim internists travel around in annoyingly large groups, like fleas, buzzing much and accomplishing little. They are notorious for one-upmanship.

"Nobody expects much from the junior residents anyway," John went on. "Just do what you're told, be prepared for every surgery, and read about every case on your service."

I thanked him and went home, feeling even worse. "Be prepared for every surgery." What did that mean? Did I have to learn how to *do* a total knee replacement before I had even seen one?

I peeled the cellophane from my brand-new copy of Campbell's *Operative Orthopedics* and began poring over the sections on total hip and knee replacements—but it was a losing battle. I would read a sentence that contained an unfamiliar word. I would look up that word only to find the definition included another word I had never heard of. I would look up *that* word and pretty soon I couldn't remember where I had started in the first place.

"So, how'd everything go?" Art asked me on Monday morning.

"Oh, fine," I said, handing him his beeper. "No problems. A couple wounds are draining a little, but everyone's okay."

Everyone, that is, except me. I had just spent forty-eight hours in hell.

Is this, I wondered, what I have to look forward to for the next four years?

# CHAPTER THREE

*July*

Having survived that first weekend, I felt a little more confident. As the days passed, Art and I began to form a routine. We met for breakfast every morning in the hospital cafeteria. Technically, only residents who had been on call the night before, or who had started work before 6:00 A.M., were entitled to free breakfast, but when Art saw me reach for my wallet at the checkout line the first day he said, "Pay no attention to that bullshit. When you work as hard as we do, breakfast is free."

The ortho residents always sat together, often taking up two or three long tables in the cafeteria. Although we would occasionally let medical students sit with us, we never allowed fleas.

I was sitting at breakfast one morning listening to the senior residents argue whether a staple from an old upper tibial osteotomy had to be removed before doing a total knee replacement. I never took part in these conversations. I was barely able to understand what they were talking about.

Down the table someone was reading the morning paper. Jack Manning, on call from the night before, was resting his head on his hand, staring bleary-eyed into space, a cold cup of coffee in front of him. Beepers were going off. Guys were hurrying away, leaving their breakfasts half-eaten. Other guys were arriving and taking their place. Several conversations were taking place at the same time.

"I'm not kidding; she kept waving her cigarette holder at Dr. Hale, telling him there was a battalion of tiny Iranian devils with poisoned pitchforks that waited 'til she fell asleep so they could start stabbing her in the groin."

"I tried to fix the lateral side first but I just couldn't reduce it. So I had to open the medial side, repair the ligament, and then go back and plate the lateral side. The damn thing took almost two hours."

Art, who wasn't interested in shoptalk, made a remark about a skirt he saw on a woman at the Depot House, Rochester's only singles bar. "Two more inches and I think I could have seen the dark side of the moon," he said.

Breakfast was Art's time to regale us with stories of his latest conquests. Handsome, witty, an excellent athlete, and an incredibly charming ladies' man, Art was a legend at Mayo. He always had some beautiful woman at his side. Although reasonably skilled as a surgeon, his work tended at times to be careless. He made no secret that his main interests were anatomic not orthopedic.

"I'm only human," he said with a sigh of helplessness. "I couldn't fight her off one more minute. Against my better judgment I finally had to give myself to her."

"Against your better judgment, huh?"

"Even the just man falls seven times a day."

"You wish."


Art and I helped Mrs. Schmidt onto the operating table. After the anesthesiologists had put her to sleep, we wrapped a tourniquet around her upper thigh, prepped and draped her, and then sent for Dr. Harding. I was excited. This would be the first total knee replacement I had ever seen.

Big John came down from the staff lounge, scrubbed in, slapped his hands together, and approached the table. He took the patient's knee in his huge hands and bent it up and down several times. He palpated both sides of the knee, then held out his hand.

"Scalpel," he said.

The scrub nurse slapped the scalpel in his hand. Before I realized what was happening, Big John had run his hand down the front of the knee, and had sliced it wide open. Layers of fat spread to either side, and despite the tourniquet, blood began to ooze from several spots.

Within sixty seconds he had opened the capsule, everted the kneecap, and exposed the joint. I could see the worn and frayed cartilage, the spurs, and the bare bone where the cartilage had eroded. Periodically Dr. Harding would cut away a glob of fat and drop it in the kick bucket next to the table.

I had pictured surgery as a series of delicate maneuvers performed with a scalpel held gently between thumb and forefinger. This procedure seemed like bloody, rapid-fire chaos. "Slash and bash," Art had called it.

When he finished exposing the joint, Dr. Harding picked up a power saw from the nurse's table and began to saw off the end of the femur. The piercing whine of the saw was unsettling, especially in light of my preconceived notions of the delicate nature of surgery.

"She's got a lot of medial compartmental erosion," John said after he finished the femoral cut. "That means we're going to have to angle our tibial cut *this* way." He grunted as he rammed a retractor into the other side of the knee.

"Here. Hold this damn thing," he said, turning to me.

I grabbed the retractor.

"Don't be afraid of it. It won't bite you," John said. "Pull hard on it. I have to be able to see the entire plateau before I make the cut."

He took the saw from the nurse, leaned to his right for better leverage, and sawed off the top of the tibia. Then he flipped over the patella and sawed off the underside of it, too.

As Art irrigated the wound with antibiotic solution, Big John turned to the scrub nurse, instructing her on what prostheses he would use. I, meanwhile, stared in fascination at the sight in front of me. Our patient's knee was filleted open. Sawed-off chunks of bone lay scattered about the field. I tried to act nonchalant, as though I were used to being surrounded by mutilated body parts.

*(Yeah, ho-hum. Just another routine dismemberment. A femur here, a kneecap there. No big deal. It's all in a day's work.)*

Art was irrigating the wound, and fluid was spilling over the side of the knee. "Hey, numb nuts," he whispered. "Suck, will you?"

I grabbed the suction and a lap sponge and began cleaning up.

John finished selecting the prosthetic components he would use. The circulating nurse opened them and dropped them on the sterile back table. John then turned to us.

"Now," he said, "the fun part."

*(So, what was the dismemberment—the boring part?)*

First he held the components against the femur and tibia, assessing the fit. He took the saw and shaved a little more off one side of the tibia.

"All right," he said, turning to the scrub nurse, "you can mix."

The nurse shook some white powder from a plastic pouch into a dish in front of her. Then she broke open a brown vial of a strong-smelling liquid and began mixing it with the powder.

Powder? Liquid? What the hell was this? Was Big John going to start sprinkling this stuff over the patient like some shaman? I half expected him to start chanting incantations. *Unga gagunga.* Was he going to promise her total consciousness on her deathbed, too? Well, at least she'd have *that* going for her.

Three minutes later the nurse told John she was ready. He took the white, creamy mixture (that I later learned was bone cement) and began applying it to the end of the bone and the undersurface of each prosthesis. He then fit the prosthesis to the bone, took a large mallet, and began banging away on it, impacting it into place.

What a strange world: blood, bone, body parts, saws, hammers. How totally different from what I had expected. We seemed more like carpenters on a construction site than surgeons in an operating room. And yet I found it incredibly exciting, and was disappointed that to everyone else it seemed so routine. I wanted them to feel as I did, that this was something extraordinary, something reverential. We had opened a human body, cut away parts of it, discarded them, put in new ones, and then closed everything up again. And in a day or two this person would be walking, her pain gone. It was incredible. I wanted to keep this awe and fascination forever. I didn't want it to ever become routine.

At 5:00 P.M., we finished our last case. I had been on call the night before, and although I had slept a few hours, the long day in the OR had worn me out. I sagged against the wall in the residents' locker room and called my wife for a ride home.

Fifteen minutes later Patti pulled up to the back entrance of Methodist Hospital. Eileen, in her car seat, was chewing on a fistful of animal crackers. She waved her free hand and garbled her hello.

I leaned in the back window, picked out a clean spot on her forehead, and kissed her. Then Patti slid over and I got behind the wheel. As I swung out of the lot, Patti laid her left hand on my forearm.

"Miss me?" she said.

I turned to her and nodded, a sleepy smile on my face. "I always miss you."

Patti was excited for me. She was a nurse, and she spoke the language. For the first few months of my residency, Patti probably knew more orthopedics than I did. She loved hearing about my work. Most young couples talk about movies or books or sports. We talked orthopedics. Constantly. In the car, over dinner, feeding the baby, doing dishes, in bed at night.

"It's amazing how much that guy bled," I said one night as I turned out the lights and reached for her.

That's where Patti drew the line. "Are we going to talk about bleeding," she said, pushing my hand away, "or are we going to—"

"Bleeding? Who cares about bleeding? Why would you want to talk about bleeding at a moment like this?"

On Friday nights those of us who weren't on call would meet, with our wives, at Tinkler's on Second Street. There would be beers, laughter—and more shoptalk.

"I'm not kidding you," Frank Wales was saying one night. "This feller was so liquored up he didn't even know his finger was missing. By the time the hand guys got him to the OR it was five A.M. I was just getting into bed when some nurse up on Seven called me to see one of Satterfield's patients, who claimed Russian spies were hiding under her bed."

"She may be on to something," Bill Chapin said as he filled our glasses from the pitcher. "I've been up on Seven, and the place is crawling with Commies."

"You're a big help. I should have had the nurses call you."

"No thanks. I was busy communicating with Martians through the fillings in my teeth. So what did you do?"

"I checked under her gol-dang bed and told her no one was there. Then she told me *I* was a Russian spy. That's when I got a psych consult."

"For you or her?"

"At that point I reckon I needed one as bad as she did."

Patti, Alice Chapin, and Linda Wales were on one side of the table chatting away, casting an occasional disapproving glance at Frank, Bill, and me if our stories got too graphic or our jokes too crude.

"Where in the hell is Manning tonight?" Frank asked. "On call?"

Bill shook his head. "No, he and Sue are at a fondue party."

"A fon—what in the Sam Hill is a fondoo party?"

"It's a party where everyone fondles everyone else," I said.

"It is not," Patti said. Like most women she could carry on three conversations and still know what is going on at all the tables around her. "A fondue party is where people gather to taste fondue. Fondue is a sort of melted cheese."

Frank looked perplexed. "Why in the hell would they want to do that?"

"It's a party, Frank," she said. "It's just a way to get together with your friends."

"So's this, and I don't need no neighbors pouring melted cheese over me neither."

"Depends on the neighbor," Bill said. "Now there are a couple of fine ladies in our neighborhood I wish would pour melted cheese over me."

"Who?" Alice said. "Leslie Wilson? As if she'd have you."

"Oh, yeah? Well, she already called and invited me to a Mazola party."

The wives laughed uproariously. "Can you see it?" Alice said, holding her sides. "Bill at a Mazola party!"

"Beats melted cheese is all I can say," Frank said.

Dr. Jonathan J. Wilhelm took a bite of his pancake, delicately wiped the corner of his mouth with his napkin, and then jerked his thumb at me. "Jesus Christ, who is this guy?"

Wilhelm was a senior resident who liked the sound of his own voice. He tended to dominate all conversations, constantly interjecting his opinion on everything. It was well known that he expected to be asked to stay on staff at Mayo when he finished his residency.

The topic at breakfast that morning was shoulder dislocations and, as usual, I just sat there and listened. They had been talking about an operation called a "Bristow." I asked Art what a Bristow was. Wilhelm couldn't believe it.

"Don't tell me this guy is an ortho resident," he said to everyone at the table. He turned to me. "Are you a medical student or a flea?"

"I'm the junior resident on Harding's service."

"*You* are an *ortho* resident?" He threw up his hands in disgust.

I was too intimidated, too shamefully aware of my own ignorance to defend myself. To his credit, Art stood up for me.

"Back off, Wilhelm. He's all right."

"All right? An ortho resident who never heard of a Bristow? Jesus Christ." He shook his head and went back to his pancakes. I was just starting to sink back into a relieved anonymity when he turned to me and said, "Did you know the hip bone is connected to the thigh bone?" He was greatly amused by this witticism and looked around the table, encouraging everyone else to join his laughter. One or two did before Art once again told Wilhelm to knock it off.

"Whatever you say, Art," Wilhelm said as the laughter subsided. "After all, you're the one who's stuck with him."

There is only so much shit one can eat. Art saw the look in my eyes and grabbed me by the elbow. "Come on, Cassius," he said. "We gotta make rounds."

Wilhelm by then had forgotten me. He was lecturing the rest of the table on the histology of ligament healing.

"Forget it," Art said, steering me away from the table. "The guy is a jerk. If the Clinic asks him to stay on staff they're out of their minds."


The Mayo work week was divided into surgery days and clinic days. We either operated all day, or we saw patients in the clinic all day. On surgery days I was the second assistant on all cases. Art would get to operate once in a while, but I did nothing more than hold retractors and write post-op orders. On clinic days I tagged along behind Art and Dr. Harding as they saw patients.

After finishing rounds one morning, Art and I made our way to the fourteenth floor of the Mayo Building. We squeezed in the door of the orthopedic residents' lounge just as three other guys were coming out. Inside, six or seven residents were reading mail, dropping off briefcases, or talking. In the corner, in an old, overstuffed armchair, a resident in a rumpled blue sport coat was sound asleep, his head lolled to the right, his mouth slightly open. A row of mail slots lined the wall on our left. Above the mail slots was a bulletin board crammed with notices from Dr. Benjamin J. ("BJ") Burke, the director of the residency program:

—"All residents are reminded that the dress code—coat and tie—remains in force on weekends. No resident is to make rounds unless in coat and tie."
—"The annual Orthopedic In-training Exam will be held on Saturday, September 23. All residents are required to take this exam."
—"Saturday morning conference is MANDATORY for all residents. NO EXCUSES!!"

As head of the residency program, Dr. Burke ran our lives. He was our lord and master, the engineer at the throttle of the train to salvation. We could not get through the program, we could not become orthopedic surgeons, unless BJ gave his blessing.

"Be careful of BJ," Art warned me. "Every year, one or two guys get on his bad side and he makes life miserable for them. He picks on them at conferences, stops them in the hall if their tie is crooked, everything. Don't piss that man off or your ass is grass."

I planned to stay as far from Dr. Burke as I could. If he found out how ignorant I was, he would bury me. "Do your job. Keep your mouth shut. Don't draw any attention to yourself" was the message I kept repeating to myself. I was, and planned to remain, the Invisible Resident.

Being the Invisible Resident on Dr. Harding's service was easy. Within a week, he must have realized how far behind I was. For that reason he did the kindest thing he could have done: he ignored me. When we made rounds it was always Art to whom he spoke. In the OR it was always Art whom he allowed to operate. I wasn't even sure if Big John knew my name—but I didn't blame him. I needed to get myself to a certain level before it was worth his while to teach me.

Of course, I had plenty of impetus to learn. It terrified me to realize my decisions could literally kill or cripple someone. Sure, there were safeguards. No one was going to hand me a scalpel on my first day. But someday my turn would come—and I'd better be ready.

I studied harder than I had ever studied before—partly because I was ashamed of my ignorance, partly because I realized that patients' health and lives would soon depend on me, and partly because I actually liked this stuff. I was falling in love with orthopedics.

Every night I took out the index cards upon which I had jotted down questions and notes. I went over them one by one, often waking at 2:00 or 3:00 A.M., my head slumped forward on the desk, drool staining the page I had been reading. I would stagger to bed and curl up next to Patti for a few hours. The next morning I would start all over again.

Art was always a bit impatient with my constant barrage of questions.

He knew if he encouraged me I would pepper him with questions all day long. But he did one thing that helped me immensely: he dumped responsibility on me. He constantly took off and left me to handle things on the service. "Heck of a deal!" was his comment on almost everything.

We were in the locker room changing into our street clothes when Art told me one of Big John's claims to fame was that he had memorized a long narrative poem about an English boy named Little Albert. An hour later, when we finished rounds, Art nudged me.

"Say, Dr. Harding, I don't think Mike here has heard *Little Albert*."

"Ah," Big John said with a smile. "You've never heard *Little Albert*?"

I confessed I had not.

He put his huge left hand on my shoulder and broke into a poem about Little Albert and his encounter with a lion. He recited it for us in a cockney accent as we stood outside the elevator on the seventh floor. His big face lit up as he glanced back and forth, eyes dancing, arms gesturing, as he related the comical story of a little boy's ill-fated visit to the zoo. The story ends with Little Albert getting eaten by the lion, after which his father philosophically observes that "what can't be helped must be endured."

I would think of that line often during the next four years.


I had six days left on Harding's service when Marvella, his secretary, called me. Prince Saleb had invited Dr. Harding, Art, and me to dinner in his suite at the Kahler Hotel. We had done a knee replacement on the prince two weeks before, and this apparently was his way of thanking us.

"Wives, too?" I asked. Patti could use a night out.

"No, Doctor, just the three of you."

Uh-oh. Pat wasn't going to be thrilled. She would have to stay home and eat Hamburger Helper with Eileen while I dined in a penthouse suite with a prince. I was already figuring out how to break the news to her when I asked Marvella, "When is the dinner?"

"Wednesday night."

I groaned. "Oh, no, not Wednesday. I'm on call." I paused, waiting for her to say, "No problem. I'll just check with the prince and see if we can make it another night." Instead she said, "That's a shame." Princes and department heads don't rearrange their schedules to accommodate junior residents.

Art told me later that the hotel catered the entire affair. It was a dinner of candlelight, crystal, and silver, served in the prince's suite on the top floor of the Kahler. The prince had rented out the entire floor for the month he stayed in Rochester.

I asked Art later if the prince had expressed any regret that I was unable to attend the dinner. Art laughed. I suppose there must be a Kuwaiti equivalent for a junior resident, and whatever it was, no prince was going to bother with him. I wondered if my declining the invitation might even have been regarded as a snub on my part. Perhaps they thought it inconceivable that Dr. Harding's "slave" would have the temerity to refuse them.

Art told me the meal went reasonably well. They ate in silence. The prince's translator stood unobtrusively several feet behind him. There was limited call for his services. The Kuwaitis were intimidated by Harding's Western aplomb, while Art and John were intimidated by the Kuwaitis' wealth.

When they were leaving, John thanked their host for a fine evening. The prince shook his hand and then spoke the only words of English any of us had ever heard from him.

"I am very much to thank you for your generous goodness on me," he said, bowing gravely. He reached over to a table upon which three small boxes were resting. He handed one to John and the other to Art.

"That last box," Art told me the next day as he stretched out his arm to show me his new Rolex watch, "was yours. Pity you couldn't make the dinner."

"He gave you a Rolex? You son of a bitch." I wadded my surgeon's cap into a ball and threw it in the corner. "While you and Big John were eating lobster and frog legs, I had four consults, a wrist fracture, and a pussed-out knee in a drug addict."

"Perhaps it's just as well," Art said. "After all, I would hate to see you become overly concerned with material things." He stabbed a piece of French toast and popped it in his mouth. "Heck of a deal!" he said.

I was just starting to feel comfortable with Dr. Harding when, in mid-August, it was time to switch services.

# CHAPTER FOUR

*August*

There were certain surgeons to whom every resident at Mayo wanted to be assigned. Tom Hale and Antonio Romero were up-and-coming stars in the department. They loved to teach, and they let their residents do a lot of operating. Fred Hastings and Garrett Freiberg were world-renowned hand surgeons. Bob Filmore was making a name for himself in the world of shoulder surgery. But the plum of them all was Mark Coventry.

Mark B. Coventry was *the* towering figure in the Department of Orthopedics at Mayo. Tall, distinguished, and white-haired, Dr. Coventry had a regal bearing that seemed both natural and deserved. So commanding was his presence that even some of the other attendings couldn't bring themselves to call him by his first name. He had pioneered a number of surgeries, and had performed the first total hip replacement in the United States. Although in the twilight of his career, Dr. Coventry was probably the most highly regarded orthopedic surgeon in the country. In mid-August I finished with Dr. Harding and started with Dr. Coventry.

From the very first day on his service, I loved being with Dr. Coventry, but I trembled to think what would have happened if I had been assigned to him *first*. He would have been appalled at my ignorance. Where Dr. Harding largely ignored me, Dr. Coventry constantly challenged me.

"What muscles are innervated by the L-4 nerve root?"

"What is a MacIntosh procedure?"

"How much does a short leg cast weigh?"

"What is the minimum acceptable hourly urine output in a post-op patient?"

Dr. Coventry demanded a lot from his residents. If there was a problem with bleeding, drainage, pain, or an abnormal lab, God help us if we didn't know about it, have an explanation for it, and have already instituted treatment for it by the time it came to his attention. These high standards were Dr. Coventry's way of reaffirming the importance of what we did. By his attitude, by his bearing, and by his insistence on perfection, he impressed upon us the seriousness of our calling.

In addition to being a renowned surgeon, Dr. Coventry was a splendid athlete. He had been a standout hockey player at Michigan in his undergraduate days. When he moved to Rochester he played semi-pro hockey for the legendary Rochester Mustangs. He told me the only reason he quit playing was because of pressure from the Clinic. After a particularly rough game, the headlines of the Rochester *Post-Bulletin* sports section read: "MUSTANGS WIN. MAYO DOCTOR IN BRAWL." That was the final straw for the Clinic administrators who objected to the unfavorable publicity. Dr. Coventry was forced to give up his hockey career.

Jim "Whit" Whitmer was the senior resident assigned to Dr. Coventry's service with me. Since Dr. Coventry insisted that his residents make "pre-round" rounds each day, Jim and I would meet every morning at six. We would see every patient on the service, and then meet Cuv, as the residents called him behind his back, for formal rounds at 7:30 A.M.

I had been on Cuv's service for two weeks and was preparing to see a patient when I found a strange-looking X-ray of the pelvis. "What the hell?" I muttered to myself. On the right side I could see a typical total hip replacement. On the left was a normal-looking hip except for wires around the greater trochanter. All hip replacements at that time involved wiring the trochanter at the conclusion of the case, but I had never seen a trochanter wired without the hip having been replaced.

I called to Jim Whitmer who had just come out of a dictating booth. "Hey, Whit, get a load of this."

He walked over. "What've you got?"

"This," I said, pointing. "Look at that left hip. It looks like—"

"Thomas Rodnovich," he said immediately.

"Thomas what?"

"Rodnovich. Thomas Rodnovich."

"You know the guy?"

"Everybody knows Thomas Rodnovich."

"Okay. Who is he? And why does he have wires in his left hip?"

Whit took a step closer. "Listen," he said, lowering his voice and looking to see if anyone else was around, "I can't believe you never heard of this case. He's a guy Cuv operated on last year. It was the last case of the day. Maybe everyone was tired, I don't know. Anyway, the case was done in a second room, and the residents somehow prepped the wrong hip. To make it worse, Stan Warczak, the junior resident, put the X-ray on the view box backward, making the right hip look like the left.

"Cuv came in after the patient had been prepped and draped. He made the incision and had just removed the greater trochanter when he sensed something was wrong. He had one of the nurses check the consent and then realized he was doing the wrong hip. Thank God all he had done was open it. He hadn't replaced the joint, but he had made an incision and had removed the trochanter on the wrong hip."

I could hardly believe such a catastrophe had happened to one of my idols, one of the gods of orthopedics.

"So what'd Cuv do?"

"He didn't say a word. He wired the trochanter back down, closed the incision, and did the other hip. Then he went out and talked to the family. He told them what happened and took all the blame himself."

Since my first day in orthopedics I had worried about what horrible things might happen if I screwed up. This story made me realize that my fears were justified. People do screw up. Terrible things do happen.

I was afraid to ask the next question. "What happened to the residents?"

"Warczak went to Cuv after the case and apologized, said he was responsible for the error and offered to resign from the residency program."

My heart was pounding. *Resign from the program!*

"Cuv heard him out and then said Stan had made a serious mistake. He should have paid more attention to what he was doing. But Cuv said *he* should have caught the mistake himself. He told Stan not to resign, but said God help him if he ever made a mistake like that again."

I had just reached over to the X-ray to point at something when Whit whipped the film off the view box.

"Hey! I wanted to—"

"Gentlemen." Cuv had come up behind us and nodded his hello. He took the X-ray out of Whit's hand and put it back on the view box.

"One should never be afraid to confront one's mistakes, Dr. Whitmer." Whit, embarrassed, nodded weakly.

"Dr. Collins, you have heard the facts of this case?"

"Yes, sir."

"And what have you concluded?"

I was about to say something patronizing about how bad breaks can happen to even the greatest of surgeons, but the look in Cuv's eye told me he didn't want bullshit. I took a deep breath.

"Well, sir, it scares the hell out of me."

"And why is that?"

"Because I've always been afraid that *I* would make some terrible mistake. This case is like my worst nightmare come true."

He nodded. "You owe it to your patients never to lose that fear, Doctor."

He reached over and straightened the X-ray, as if giving it permission to beam out his error to the whole world.

"This," he said, "is what happens from a lack of vigilance on the part of the surgeon." I could tell he was speaking as much to himself as to us. "Everything that happens in that operating room is your responsibility. Everything. On the operating table lies an unconscious, helpless patient who has placed his confidence and trust in *you*—not in the resident, not in the anesthesiologist, not in the institution, but in you."

His shoulders sagged. He was visibly shaken. Even a year later, he was still suffering from what had happened that day. Whit and I looked at each other. There was nothing we could do to comfort him. Any words mere residents could say would only make it worse.

"Gentlemen," he told us, "you will find that you can learn much more about yourself from your failures than from your successes."

If there had been any doubt in my mind about going into orthopedics it was removed on Mark Coventry's service. He showed me how rewarding and fulfilling life as a surgeon could be.

I had chosen surgery instead of internal medicine because I wanted to *do* things. Too often internists seemed interested only in the process of discovery. They wanted to *learn* things. What was the diagnosis? What caused it? The emphasis was always on examining and discerning, not fixing. "Internists diagnose and surgeons treat" is the old expression. Of course, internists put it another way: internists think; surgeons act.

Back then, orthopedic surgeons had the unfair reputation of being the dummies of the medical profession. We were the not-very-bright plodders who fixed broken things. Orthopods, so the internists claimed, were usually ex-jocks who were "strong as an ox and twice as smart."

I attended Loyola Stritch School of Medicine in Chicago. Every year on the feast of St. Luke, the patron saint of physicians, the school held a big dinner. Skits were performed lampooning each specialty. Jokes would be made about anesthesiologists passing gas. The obstetrician would wear a catcher's mitt. The pediatrician would have a lollipop in her mouth. And always, the orthopod would be some big, dumb guy with a tool belt strapped to his waist. His only dialogue would be something like "Bone broke. Me fix."

Despite the jokes about orthopedics, I felt drawn to it. I had always liked to work with my hands. As a child, I constructed models and forts and castles. I enjoyed building things, starting with nothing and making it into something.

On Dr. Coventry's service everything came together. He showed me the nobility of our calling. He showed me how seriously we must take our responsibilities. But, above all, he showed me how wonderful it felt to do something for others.

I learned from Dr. Coventry to enjoy the time we spent in the clinic. Like most orthopods I preferred the operating room to the clinic. The OR was where our hearts lay. That's where great things were done. What happened in the clinic always seemed a preparation for, or a postscript to, what we did in the OR.

But there was a difference with Cuv. Going to the clinic with him was a heady experience. Every day, in almost every room, were people he had helped, people who were so incredibly grateful to him. I couldn't get over it. Just thinking that someday I might be able to accomplish similar things made me giddy.

Frank, Jack, and Bill were jealous that I got to be with Cuv.

"So what's he like?" Jack asked me one Friday night at Tinkler's.

"Well, he's a no-bullshit kind of guy," I said. "He's always asking you questions, always checking to be sure you haven't overlooked something. He seems kind of cold and aloof when you first meet him, but he grows on you. What's amazing is seeing him with patients. He's all business when he examines them; but when it's time to sit down and talk, he's a different guy. All the sternness is gone. You can feel his warmth, how genuine he is."

I know Cuv must have had his failures, but I don't recall ever seeing one. Even a guy like Thomas Rodnovich, upon whom Cuv had made a mistake, certainly could not be classified as a failure. All his pre-operative pain was gone, and he was delighted with Cuv and his care.


Whit and I had positioned, prepped, and draped Mrs. Bergmann for her total hip operation. We waited at the OR table while Gladys, the nurse who always worked with Dr. Coventry, gowned and gloved him. He approached the table with an air of quiet confidence.

He nodded good morning to Whit and me, then silently held out his hand. Gladys placed the scalpel in it. "Dr. Collins," Cuv announced in his stern voice, "will make the incision." He handed the scalpel to me.

I was stunned—thrilled, but stunned. I hadn't expected it. Tired from being up all night, I was prepared for another routine surgery. I had been working with Dr. Coventry for almost six weeks. I knew the answers to all his pet questions, and was prepared for a nice, relaxing ride watching Whit and Cuv work while I mindlessly assisted. Suddenly I could feel my heart pounding. I had never made an incision before. I had never "cut."

As residents, even junior residents, we wanted to operate. That's what surgeons do—they operate. And until we got to pick up a scalpel and cut it was hard to think of ourselves as real surgeons.

Sometimes at the beginning of a case, while we waited for the attending surgeon to scrub in, we would stare at that gleaming steel blade lying on the Mayo stand. We longed to take it in our hands. We craved the power and skill it represented. The scalpel was a symbol of that other world that was waiting for us, the world of operating rooms and surgery, the world of "hot lights and cold steel," as the older guys called it.

The attendings knew that every resident wanted to do every case. At the beginning of the quarter, the attending would observe his senior resident, assessing his competence and confidence, judging his ability to operate. If the resident seemed to know what he was doing, if he answered anatomical questions correctly, if he was attentive and respectful, the attending would usually turn over more and more cases to him.

As junior residents we dreamed of someday doing our first total hip or rotator cuff repair, but we knew it wasn't going to happen until we paid our dues working the suction and the cautery, cutting sutures and maybe sewing the skin. Frank and Jack had already done a couple minor procedures. So far Bill and I had never even touched a scalpel.

Frank wasn't very sympathetic. "They don't make scalpels with training wheels," he said. "Why you two dang fools are more likely to cut yourselves than the patient."

I had sutured many times, had closed many lacerations, and now, finally, I was being given my chance to cut.

Cuv stepped back and motioned for me to assume the head surgeon's position. Gladys, Cuv, Whit, the two anesthesiologists, and the circulators all stood watching. I could see Whit's eyes smiling in amusement as he watched my uncertainty.

"Well, Doctor?" Cuv said.

I laid down the scalpel and felt the hip, searching for the landmarks I would use to make the incision.

Is that the greater trochanter? I thought in panic. She was fat, and it was hard to tell. I palpated her skin one more time before I took the skin marker from Gladys and drew a long purple line indicating where I would make my incision.

Cuv felt the hip and nodded his approval. I held out my trembling hand to Gladys who was obviously enjoying my discomfort. "Scalpel, Doctor," she said.

Holding the scalpel gingerly in my fingertips, I prepared to make the incision.

"Not like that!" Dr. Coventry boomed in irritation. "You don't hold it like a pencil. Put it in your hand and hold it like a man." He took the scalpel from me and demonstrated, holding the scalpel deep in his palm.

Intimidated, feeling like I was failing my first big test, I took the scalpel and once again approached the wound. I glanced briefly at Cuv for reassurance, but his eyes peered unwaveringly from above his blue mask and told me nothing. I took a deep breath, brought my hand forward, then drew the scalpel down the long purple mark. I took my hand away and seven pair of eyes looked expectantly at what I had done. A tiny, superficial scratch that was scarcely deep enough to draw blood was etched along the length of the hip.

"What was that?" Cuv grated. I could see Whit laughing from behind Cuv's shoulder. "At this rate we'll be here all day. Push on that thing and make a decent incision."

I grasped the knife, then realized I was holding it like a pencil again. I shifted it back, deeper in my palm. I brought my hand back up to the top of the mark and pushed with what seemed like reckless force. Once again I brought my hand down the length of the purple mark, afraid that at any moment my hand might plunge into the depths of the wound and cut several arteries and nerves.

We all looked again. This time I had at least incised down to the subcutaneous tissue.

"Very nice, Doctor," Whit murmured in mock approval. Cuv stood straight and still, saying nothing. I leaned forward to proceed.

"Deep knife," Cuv corrected.

Since the base of hair follicles may still harbor bacteria even after the skin has been scrubbed, the knife that is used to make the skin incision is considered to be contaminated. Once the incision is made, the "skin knife" is discarded in favor of the sterile "deep knife." I turned to Gladys who was already waiting with the correct knife.

Down through the greasy yellow fat I drew my scalpeled hand. Whit and Cuv held the Israel retractors as I worked my way deeper and deeper. I could tell they were growing impatient. I told myself there were no significant anatomical structures in the area. I wanted to go faster, but I couldn't. It was all too new. I was terrified that at any moment I might find myself staring in horror at the severed ends of the sciatic nerve (which I knew was nowhere near me).

Cuv restrained himself admirably. What was taking me ten minutes would have taken him thirty seconds, yet he assisted me silently and competently, pulling the wall of yellow fat back from the operative field, and using the suction to point my way.

Finally I reached the fascia overlying the hip. Cuv tapped the fascia with the suction. "Can you identify this structure, Doctor?"

"That is the tensor fascia lata."

He gently edged me over. "And directly below it is . . .?"

"The vastus lateralis muscle."

Cuv nodded, handed me the Israel retractor, and picked up the scalpel. "What is the innervation of the vastus?" he asked as he incised the fascia in one delicate stroke.

I was back to being a junior resident. My time in the spotlight had ended. This dog had had his day. I told Cuv the femoral nerve innervated the vastus. He nodded approvingly and said, "Well done, Doctor."

Cuv had thrown me a crumb. He let me open. He had done the same for countless junior residents before me. It was a moment he probably forgot within a week, but for me that crumb was a gourmet feast. I had held a scalpel in my hand and I had cut.

I was a surgeon.

# CHAPTER FIVE

*September*

The ERSS. Even the name had a dark, sinister resonance.

On September 26 I completed my six weeks with Dr. Coventry and was assigned to the Emergency Room Surgical Service at St. Mary's Hospital. Every car crash, every farm injury, every gunshot wound—every major trauma in southeast Minnesota was brought to St. Mary's and cared for by the ERSS.

There were three general surgery junior residents assigned to the ERSS with me: Mac Self, Rollie Whitfield, and Jerry Washburn. The attending surgeon of the ERSS was Dr. Joe Stradlack. Joe was an archetypal, frenetic trauma surgeon who constantly struggled with his inability to speak as rapidly as he thought. When excited, he could hardly finish one word before starting the next.

I had heard one of the other residents at breakfast doing an imitation of Joe: "Trauma big time gotta move on this guy full code type-and-cross cut-down crack his chest get the lines in subclavian large-bore pump the fluid where the hell is anesthesia?"

Joe was only a few years out of his residency but was fiercely dedicated to teaching residents and to improving the quality of care provided in the Mayo emergency rooms. The residents loved him. I was sorry to leave Dr. Coventry, but I couldn't wait to get in the trenches with Joe Stradlack and "go to war."

On our first morning on ERSS we reported to the tiny conference room next to the ER. Joe Stradlack filled us in on our responsibilities.

"You junior residents will be on call every other night. That means"— he consulted the paper in front of him—"Collins and Whitfield, you are on tonight; and"—another glance at the paper—"Self and Washburn, you are on tomorrow."

On the nights we weren't on call, Joe said, we could go home; but if there were emergencies we might be called back in.

Mac, Jerry, Rollie, and I looked at the four junior residents who were just finishing their stint on the ERSS. Three of them were already sprawled asleep in their chairs. The fourth, disheveled and unshaven, was holding a cup of coffee on his lap and staring ahead unseeingly.

*"Morituri te salutant,"* Mac whispered to me.

*"Semper ubi, sub ubi,"* I replied.

A week later, when we hadn't had one good night's sleep among the four of us, Mac called us together.

"Look," he said, "this is bullshit. I don't want to spend the rest of my time on ERSS being here every goddamn day and night."

Rollie rubbed a hand across the stubble on his chin. "Neither do I," he said with a loud yawn, "but since when does it matter what we want? We're slaves, remember?"

"The hell we are," he said. "I have an idea." He took the cup of coffee from Rollie's hand and set it on the table. "Listen to me." He pointed at Rollie and me. "I swear to you, I swear to God, that from now on, when I am on call and you two are at home, I will not let them call you back in. Whatever it takes, I'll do it. Even if I have to lock Joe Stradlack in the morgue, I will not let him call you back in." I could see the determination on his face and I knew what he had in mind.

I nodded. "And we do the same for you."

"You got it."

Like little kids forming a secret club, we solemnly shook hands and swore we would never allow the two guys at home to be called back in.

Sure enough, that night when Rollie and I went home, we weren't called back in. We slept all night and didn't go back to the hospital until 6:30 the following morning. Later, when Mac and Jerry were going off duty, I looked up from the face I was suturing and waved a sterile hand at them. "Go home," I said. "I'll see you tomorrow."

It worked. We made it work. We did whatever it took to cover for each other. We made up stories. We worked twice as hard. But our best resource was the shameless commandeering of medical students.


Joe Stradlack was rushing a lady with a hot gallbladder up to the OR for an emergency cholecystectomy.

"Mike," he called, "come on. I'm going to need you to assist."

I held up my gloved hands. "I can't. I'm sewing up a guy's leg."

"Then call Mac or Jerry from home."

No way, I thought.

I stripped off my gloves and sprinted into the hall. A kid with an armful of books was walking by. "Are you a medical student?" I asked.

"Um, yes," came the startled response.

"Thank God," I said. "We have an emergency in the ER and we need your help." I grabbed his arm in a way that would dispel any doubts he had about his ability to refuse my "request."

"Do you know how to scrub?" I asked.

"Well, I—"

"Good."

I took his books from him and tossed them on a chair. "Get into the locker room and change, then get up to OR 4. They need you right away. Emergency."

He stood there befuddled. "But I've got a biochem quiz in ten minutes."

I pointed to the locker room. "Get going. Do you want her to die?"

He looked at his books, looked at me, and then sprinted for the locker room.

I pitied the poor kid. I knew he would be stuck with a big old Deaver retractor in both hands trying to pull the liver and several inches of fat out of the way while Joe dug around, trying to take out the gallbladder.

"The Right Upper Quadrant Man," we called the guy holding the Deaver. He was always the guy with the lowest seniority. His retractor would be positioned by the head surgeon. The student would be told to grasp the retractor with two hands and then step back slightly. The surgeon and his first assistant would then wedge themselves in front of him to perform the surgery. The poor student couldn't see a thing except the back of the surgeons' gowns. During the operation, one of the surgeons might amuse himself by firing a question over his shoulder: "Can you identify this structure?"

The student wouldn't know what to say. "I, uh—"

"No, not that one, this one."

"I can't really—"

"Try paying a little more attention."

"Yes, sir," he would mumble. Asshole, he would think.


I pulled in the driveway at home, shut off the engine, and slumped back, too tired to get out of the car. Even though I was no longer getting called back into the hospital on my night off, I was still working thirty to thirty-six hours in a row, followed by twelve to eighteen hours off. When I wasn't working, all I wanted to do was sleep.

I sat in the car, head back, eyes closed for several minutes. Finally I sighed, picked up my shaving kit, heaved myself out of the front seat, and went in the back door.

Eileen, as usual, was penned in the kitchen. "Daddy!" she called as she trotted to me with her arms outstretched. I picked her up and nuzzled my face into her neck. She gurgled in delight. I carried her over to the sink where Patti was standing.

"Hey, hon," I said. I shifted Eileen to the other hip and leaned forward to give Patti a kiss. She was pregnant with our second child, and must have found it difficult caring for Eileen and taking care of the house without any help from me. But I didn't know. Most of the time I was too tired to even ask.

"Hi, you." She looked me up and down and smiled sympathetically. "How was your day, er, night?"

"Ah, okay, I guess." Eileen began squirming so I put her down. "We got another hunting accident in last night—a kid shot in the belly by his brother who thought he was a deer."

"Let me guess. The brother had a few brewskis."

"Nope. Schnapps. He just wanted to ward off the chill."

"So is the kid going to make it?"

"Well, it's a miracle he didn't bleed out before they got him to us. His brother wadded up a flannel shirt and jammed it into the hole in his belly. That probably saved his life." I tried to remember what happened next. "We took him to the OR. Joe was going to take out part of his liver or bowel or something," I said slowly, "but then I had to do a cut-down on some guy in the ER, so I don't know if the kid made it or not." I reached over and took a carrot from the cutting board. "I'll have to ask Jerry about it tomorrow."

I didn't even know if he lived or died. What was the matter with me? Was I becoming so calloused I didn't care about my patients?

I took some silverware from the drawer and began setting the table.

"So, how are you feeling?" I asked Patti.

"Tired, but fine. And," she said, turning to me, "I saw the doctor today. He says the baby is doing great."

I smiled at her. "That's awesome. Did you get a nap?"

"Yes, thank God. When I put Eileen down for her nap I laid down for an hour, too."

"Speaking of lying down for an hour, I thought I'd—"

"Oh, Mike, don't. Dinner'll be ready in twenty minutes. If you lay down I'll never get you up. Just sit here with me until dinner's ready. Please?"

She pushed me into a chair, then opened the refrigerator. "Here," she said, "have a beer and engage me in some scintillating conversation."

I took a sip of beer. It felt good just to sit there . . .

"Mike!"

My head snapped up. "Huh? Sorry."

"Come on, hon. Talk to me. I'm desperate. I have no one to talk to all day except Eileen." She came over and started massaging my shoulders. "Tell me about that drunk guy from Friday, the one who drove his golf cart off the bridge. Has he gone home yet?"

I didn't want to talk about the drunk guy. I didn't want to talk about anything. I didn't want to drink beer or eat or watch TV either. I just wanted to sleep.

The next thing I knew Patti was jabbing me in the ribs. "Here's your dinner," she said, slamming a plate in front of me.

What I should have said at that moment was, "Patti, although I am terribly tired, you are the most important thing in my life. I apologize for seeming so disinterested, but in a few weeks I will be off ERSS and our life will get back to normal."

What I actually said was, "Patti, I . . . uh . . . just . . ." I couldn't remember what I wanted to say next. I ate my dinner and went to bed.


The next day at morning report, I looked for Jerry. I wanted to ask him about the kid who got shot. I couldn't even remember his name. Jeff something.

In front of the room, one of the senior residents was giving report on a couple that had been brought in from a car crash on I-90. "Joe's up in surgery with the husband. He's got a ruptured spleen and a flail chest," he said. "The wife's in CT. She's stable, but she's got a femoral shaft fracture and a big scalp laceration. Her belly tap was negative."

I was half listening. I wanted to talk to Jerry about the kid. Unfortunately, Jerry was on the floor, propped up against the crash cart, sound asleep.

As usual the room was packed with everyone who was coming on, everyone who was going off, plus techs, nurses, and medical students. I excused myself and pushed over to Mac.

"Mac, how's the kid with the gunshot wound?"

He frowned. "Svendsen, the one from Wayzata?"

"No, the one who came in yesterday. The one whose brother shot him."

"Oh, yeah, that kid." He rubbed his forehead. "Joe took out half his liver. We couldn't get the damned thing to stop bleeding. Hell, we must have given him twenty units of blood in the OR. Then platelets, fresh frozen, everything." He cupped his hands around his coffee and closed his eyes.

"So how is he?" I asked impatiently.

Mac's head jerked upright again. He took a sip of his coffee. "Well, he made it through surgery. I don't know what happened after that. Ask Jerry. He's been up in ICU with him. I've been down here. We had a special on drunks last night. In fact, I personally established an all-time Mayo Clinic record. I had no less than four drunks tell me they were going to beat the shit out of me as soon as they got out of here."

"Did you tell them they'd have to get in line?"

"No, jerkoff, I gave 'em your home phone number and told them you said they were a bunch of pussies and you could kick their ass."


It was ten o'clock before I could get to the ICU to check on the kid. I looked at the chart next to his bed. Larson, that was his name. Jeff Larson.

His eyes were closed. I reached over his IV lines and touched him on the shoulder. "Hey, Jeff," I said. He didn't respond.

I started leafing through his chart. We were having trouble maintaining his pressure. His urine output was negligible. His lytes and labs were all over the place: SGOT up, hemoglobin down, amylase up, sodium down, BUN up, potassium down.

I looked at his belly and saw greenish-brown fluid seeping through the gauze. I wasn't sure what it was—blood, bile, betadine, pus, feces? I had just finished changing the dressings when Joe Stradlack came in. I gestured questioningly at the drainage.

"Bile," he said, "and a little blood, probably." We stepped into the hall. Joe told me he didn't think the kid was going to make it. "He had a hole the size of my fist right through his belly—liver, gallbladder, colon, intestines, everything. I don't know how he didn't bleed to death right there in the woods."

We went out to talk to Jeff's family. The parents, an older couple with their arms around each other, listened quietly. Jeff's brother, the one who shot him, stood off to the side. He hadn't left the hospital since they brought Jeff in. He was sober now, and I could see the anguish in his red-rimmed eyes.

We'd better be careful with him, I thought. He's one who could go home and shoot himself when this is all over.

When Joe finished laying out the facts for the family I tried to help the brother. "You saved him," I said. "Sticking that shirt in his wound kept him from bleeding to death. We never would have had a chance with him if it hadn't been for you."

He said nothing. He just shook his head and walked away.

I turned to his father. "Mr. Larson, there isn't a lot you can do for Jeff, but your other son . . ." I nodded at the brother, standing alone at the end of the room, his back to us, looking out the window. "Accidents happen," I said. "It's no one's fault. Your son, well, he's taking this pretty hard."

The old man held up a hand, and exhaled in disgust. Maybe he thought his son should take it hard. Maybe he blamed him for what happened to Jeff.

But I wasn't going to let it go. Two weeks before we had taken care of a man who lost control of his car and hit a little girl. He had just a few cuts and bruises. The girl, however, was seriously injured. We weren't sure she was going to survive.

The man was wracked with guilt. Although his blood alcohol was below the level of legal intoxication, he had been drinking, and had been given a ticket for negligent driving. He blamed himself for everything. He kept asking us if the girl was going to be okay. We assured him we'd do everything we could for her. But he continued to pace around, agitated and distraught. We finally got his cuts cleaned and dressed, and sent him home. Three hours later the paramedics brought him back. He had blown his brains out.

Jeff's brother had that same haunted look in his eyes. I tried to spell it out as clearly as I could for the father. "Look, Mr. Larson," I said, "if you don't want another tragedy on your hands, you go to your son and tell him that you know it was an accident and you forgive him."

The old man finally understood what I was saying. He looked shocked and then terrified. "Oh, Jesus," he muttered. He turned, walked directly over to his son, and began speaking forcefully. After a minute, the son, who had been staring at the ground the whole time, lifted his head and looked at his father. They hesitated for a moment, then took a step forward, embraced, and began clapping each other gently on the back.

I was with Jeff when he died later that night. It was the first time I had ever seen someone die, and it wasn't what I expected. It was so matter-of-fact, so ordinary. His pressure dropped, his heart quit, and he died. That was it. I stood there waiting for something momentous to happen, for someone to say something profound, but there was nothing. The nurse sighed and turned off the IV, the respiratory tech disconnected the oxygen, and the secretary called the morgue.

I still had the childish notion that since *my* life was so important, *all* lives were so important. Since *my* death would be so cataclysmic, *all* deaths would be so cataclysmic. When I saw that nothing happened when Jeff died, I realized that nothing would happen when I died. Life went on without Jeff Larson, and life would go on without Mike Collins. The nurse would sigh and turn off the IV, the respiratory tech would disconnect the oxygen, and the secretary would call the morgue.

I wondered if all the truths I would learn in medicine would be this difficult to ignore.

# CHAPTER SIX

*October*

Not every patient we cared for on ERSS had major trauma. Vern was a forty-year-old guy with a bushy red mustache and a fishhook up his nose. He had been fishing on Lake Pepin when his brother's cast snagged him. The hook had embedded itself somewhere deep inside the nose. The eye of the hook, with a small monofilament knot still attached to it, glittered in the entrance to the left nostril.

Joe Stradlack thought this would be an excellent case for a junior resident to tackle. "If you do a good job," he said, "we may let you lance a rectal abscess sometime."

A rectal abscess. Oh, gee, could I?

I numbed up Vern's nose, but after that everything seemed to conspire against me: the mustache, the lighting, the exposure, the bleeding. I shaved away part of the mustache, but still couldn't see the tip of the hook. My plan was to use a small wire-cutter to snip the shaft, then I would try to wiggle the hook free. If I could spread the nostril a little wider I might be able to see better.

I had an idea. I turned to one of the nurses. "Get me a pediatric vaginal speculum."

"Bull *shit*!" Vern bellowed from under the drapes.

"Vern, relax. It's been cleaned and sterilized. It's perfectly fine."

"I don't care what it is. You're not sticking one of those things in *my* nose."

So, did he want to go through the rest of his life with a fishhook up his nose?

"Fine," I said. I turned back to the nurse. "Get me the nostril dilator."

She stared at me uncomprehendingly. "There's no such—"

"You know. The chromium-handled, fishhook-extracting nostril dilator?" I did everything but wink at her.

"Oh," she said. "Oh, yes, the nostril dilator."

She opened the gyne cart and handed me an instrument.

Fifteen minutes later I had irrigated away enough blood and had dilated the nostril enough to snip the shaft of the hook. Now I just had to tease the barbed point out of the tissue. It was not going well. Vern was having a hard time holding still. Perhaps the fact that he had a vaginal speculum and half a hardware store stuffed up his nose was part of the problem.

"How buch logger is diss gudda take, Doc?"

"Hang in there, Vern. I just about have it."

"Dat's what you said tweddy bidutes ago."

"Have you ever tried to take a fishhook out of someone's nose?"

Finally, I slid a small, curved-needle holder deep into the nostril. I grasped the hook and pushed it through the tissue and out the skin of the nose. I reached around and pulled the hook out.

Vern let out a hideous scream and leaped off the cart. "Ow! Fuckin-A! Oh, my nose! Jesus Christ! Fer da love a' Cry-yi!" The vaginal speculum was still dangling from his nose. I must have hit a small artery because bright red blood was gushing from both inside and outside Vern's nose.

"Vern, would you please—"

"I'm outta here," he said. "I'm the fuck outta here."

"Vern, we're all done. I just want to—"

"Fuckin' right you're all done." He ripped the sterile drape off his chest and started walking to the door.

"You can't leave. You've still got the—"

He reached up and grabbed the bloody speculum and yanked it out of his nose. He stared at the speculum, his eyes narrowing. "It *is*," he said. "It is one of those things." He gave me a look of disgust, threw the speculum in the corner, and stomped out the door just as Joe Stradlack came back.

"Collins," he said, "what the hell's going on here?"

"Mr. Merven's not very happy. Apparently he has more pressing business elsewhere. I got the fishhook out, though." I held it up for him.

"Took you long enough," he said, looking at his watch.

I shrugged my shoulders and began peeling off my gloves. "So, does this mean I'm not going to get to lance any rectal abscesses?"

Twelve hours later I was assisting one of the senior residents on an appendectomy. Halfway through the case we were told there was an emergency in the ER. The senior resident let me close while he headed down to help. I finished up, brought the patient to the recovery room, and wrote the post-op orders. Then I spoke with her parents, letting them know everything had gone well. I took a minute to splash a little water on my face and then went back to the ER.

The place was packed. There must have been fifteen people crowded around a cart working on a young woman. I asked Amy Watkins, one of the nurses, what was going on.

"She ruptured an artery or something. No one knows," Amy said. "She was in full arrest when she got here."

"How long have they been working on her?"

"Long time," she said. "The paramedics started CPR on the scene and we have been doing it for almost half an hour now."

That meant her chances were poor. I glanced over at her. She was a young woman, about my age. Her gray face was partially obscured by the ET tube and the Ambu bag they were using to breathe for her.

"Who are all these people?" I asked, nodding at the crowd.

"Well, besides ERSS and the code team they have the Neonatal team here, too."

"Neo? What are *they* doing here?"

"She's forty weeks pregnant."

"Jesus," I murmured.

Joe Stradlack was standing at the foot of the cart running the code. The patient had three or four lines going in her. A team of anesthesiologists at her head was bagging her. Rollie Whitfield was doing chest compressions.

Suddenly Joe turned and looked into the crowd at the foot of the cart. "Is Neo here?" he asked.

"Yes," one of the residents answered. She looked awfully young.

"Who are you?"

"Mary Whithers, Neonatal ICU."

"What are the baby's chances?" Joe asked her. He knew damn well what the baby's chances were. I think he just wanted to see what sort of resident he was dealing with, whether he could trust her with what was to come.

"Well," she answered falteringly, "even under the best of circumstances CPR will not adequately oxygenate the fetus."

"So?"

"So the sooner you can deliver it the better—at least as far as the fetus is concerned."

Joe nodded and turned back to the woman in front of him.

Oh, God, I thought. I know what he must be thinking. CPR had by then been going on for over half an hour. The woman had no rhythm. Joe had to make a decision. If he continued CPR, the baby had no chance. If he stopped CPR and took the child by C-section, the mother had no chance.

He hesitated just a moment, then grabbed a small cup of betadine, splashed it on the abdomen, and picked up a scalpel. He slashed once, twice, three times, spread apart the gaping wound with his hands, reached in, and pulled out a perfectly formed, full-term baby. He cut and clamped the cord, then handed the child to Mary Whithers.

Now everything changed. Now instead of being the anonymous observer in the back of the crowd, Mary was the center of attention. Everyone stopped and watched to see what she could do. Nurses, surgeons, anesthesiologists, and techs all stared at the child she now held in her hands.

The child, a girl, was still warm and slippery. Mary set her down, slipped an ET tube down her throat, and had one of the nurses begin bagging her.

"Does anyone else know how to do neonatal CPR?" she shouted. One of the anesthesiologists said he knew, so she let him take over the chest compressions. Joe did a cut-down on the child's arm and got a large-bore IV going. Mary very calmly and systematically began giving resuscitation orders. She tried everything; she gave every possible drug, but the baby didn't respond. Finally, in desperation, Mary tried intracardiac epinephrine.

Even when it became obvious that there was nothing else to do, she couldn't bring herself to stop. This baby was not a premie. She was a full-term, perfectly developed baby, the kind you see on the cover of baby magazines. This was supposed to be the beginning of her life, not the end.

After another ten minutes Joe Stradlack finally laid a hand on her shoulder. "Good job, Mary," he said. "There was nothing we could do. We got them too late."

Mary looked at him, too beaten to speak. She hung her head and let her hands dangle limply at her side.

As everyone started to drift away, I glanced at the still, gray figure of the mother lying on the gurney. The overhead lights were still trained on her. Someone had tossed a sheet over the lower half of her body. The ET tube dangled limply from the side of her mouth. Then I saw that one of the nurses had brought the baby over and laid her next to her mother. The two of them lay there side by side. I tore my eyes away. I couldn't look anymore.

What the hell kind of world is this? I thought.

I looked at the tray littered with used syringes, needles, vials of meds, bloodstained 4×4s, scalpels, and hemostats: the paraphernalia of futility.

In the corner of the room Mary Whithers was standing by herself trying not to cry.

I thought Joe gestured to me to follow him. I don't know, maybe he didn't. I wouldn't have followed him if I had known where he was going. This was the part I couldn't handle, the human part. Joe had to go tell a young husband we had failed. His wife and his baby were dead.

Joe took the husband's hand, and struggled to find words. "I . . . I'm so sorry to tell you that . . ."

He said we were sorry. We were heartbroken. We had tried everything. We would have done anything. Everything that could be done had been done. And then the man thanked us. He shook our hands, even mine—I, who had done nothing. This was too much. I wasn't ready to be thanked. I wanted to punch myself, or the world, or someone. *Mothers and babies shouldn't die!*

I let the man shake my hand, and then I walked out of the ER. I leaned against the wall rubbing my left hand over my right, overwhelmed by what had just happened. It was quarter to seven. The halls were full of clean, fresh, young doctors and nurses, reporting for duty. They had been sleeping all night, had gotten up, showered, and come into work. For them it was the beginning of a new day. For me it was still one long yesterday.

I had a few minutes before morning report. I thought I'd better go check on that girl whose appendix we had taken out. Numbly, I waited for the elevator. When I got in, Jack Manning, showered, shaved, and bright-eyed, was standing there. He smiled and said hello. He could see I had been on call.

"Hey, bud," he said. "How was your night?"

# CHAPTER SEVEN

*November*

It was my last week on ERSS. I dragged myself in the back door, not watching where I was going. Eileen, who had heard the car pull into the garage, was sitting on the floor waiting for me. I stepped on her foot, stumbled forward, and whacked my shin against a chair.

"Goddamn it," I barked as Eileen started to cry.

"You stepped on her," Patti said, rushing to pick her up.

I sat down and rubbed my shin. "What the hell was she doing right inside the door anyway?"

"She was waiting for *you*. She hasn't seen you in two days. And then you go and step on the poor thing." She turned to Eileen and began stroking her hair. "It's okay, sweetie. It's okay." Eileen, sobbing, shoulders shaking, was clinging to Patti's neck.

I ran a hand across my face. I didn't need this. I had managed only a half hour of sleep the night before and had been second-assisting at some boring-as-hell belly surgery since 10:00 A.M. I wanted to walk in the back door of my house and be left alone. I wanted peace, quiet, no one telling me what to do, no beeper, no demands. I wanted to turn off my brain and my senses.

Jesus Christ, I thought. Can't I get two seconds' peace in my own house? My kid is screaming. My wife is bitching. I don't need this. I get enough of it all day and all night at work.

Six weeks on ERSS had taken a lot out of me. I had witnessed a seemingly endless procession of gunshot wounds, amputations, ruptured bowels, car crashes—and death. Yes, I had seen a lot of death. But I didn't dwell on it. Dwelling on death wasn't pragmatic, and above all I had learned to be pragmatic. Things that would have appalled me two months before now seemed routine. There were so many tragedies, and I was so busy, so tired. Resigned indifference was the only way I could keep myself from being swallowed up.

I had learned to ignore everything but the job in front of me. I had been a terrible husband, a terrible father. I was rarely home, and when I was, I had no patience for anything, no energy for anything, no interest in anything.

I was standing in the ICU, at the foot of the bed of a young girl with a severe head injury. I couldn't remember how she was injured. Car accident maybe—or was it a fall? I was watching helplessly as her temperature rose from 101 to 102 to 103. Her fever was not due to infection. It was due to severe damage to the thermoregulatory center of the brain stem.

I had packed her in ice. I had performed cool gastric lavages. I had done everything I could think of, but her temp still climbed: 104, 105. If her temperature rose much higher her chances of survival were minimal— and if she did survive, she would be a vegetable. The brain can't take temperatures that high.

Jesus Christ, I thought, she's only twenty. What the hell is wrong with me that I can't stop this?

I stood there squeezing the chart as her temp rose to 106, 107.

Joe Stradlack came by, annoyed that I was spending so much time with a patient who had no hope of surviving. But he could see I was having a hard time with this.

"Mike, we did all we could. She just . . . Well, sometimes there's just too much trauma." He patted me on the shoulder, took the chart from my hand, and dropped it in the rack at the foot of the bed. "Come on," he said gently, "we need you back in the ER."

Joe had his bearings about him. I did not. Joe knew when to fight and how to fight and when to quit fighting. He knew just how much of himself he could afford to pour into each case. But I knew none of that. I was still used to winning every fight, and those past few weeks on the ERSS were killing me.

I suddenly realized how unprepared I was for all this. Oh, I had to have been sharp to get a residency at the Mayo Clinic. I knew my anatomy and physiology. I did well on the National Boards. I had wonderful letters of recommendation from my deans. I came very well trained for the cognitive aspects of my work, but there was no training for the emotional aspects. Letters and board scores could never prepare me to lose the struggle to save a pregnant woman and her baby, or to watch a twenty-year-old girl slowly fry her brain.

No, I was not prepared for such things, and they were beginning to rip me apart. How, I wondered, can life go on? How can my fellow residents and I continue to smile, to cut the lawn on our day off, to have children?

Of course, it would have been easier if we didn't care, and sometimes we actually pretended we didn't. We would try to do our job and be detached. But we didn't go into medicine to be detached. We went into medicine because we cared. But caring kept bringing us pain and frustration and anguish.

We had been training for years to become surgeons. We had excelled in college. We had excelled in medical school. Our lives had been one success after another until we woke up one day, and there we were, surgical residents at the world-famous Mayo Clinic. It was all so perfect. But before we could congratulate ourselves, scarcely before we learned where the surgeons' locker room was, we discovered this was a profession that, like no other, quickly and ruthlessly and uncaringly proclaimed we were *not* perfect. People came to us with head injuries—and we couldn't help them. People came to us with gunshot wounds—and we couldn't heal them. People came to us with ruptured arteries—and we couldn't save them.

We kept confronting these terrible problems, and we kept failing, again and again and again—we, who had always succeeded, who had always known what to do, who had always been so sure of ourselves. Never before had we attempted anything so important, and never before had we failed so miserably.

Oh, sure, we tried to let conventional wisdom shield us. "Look," we'd tell ourselves, "you did exactly the right thing, exactly what the textbooks say you should do. Just because she died doesn't mean it was your fault."

That's what we'd tell ourselves, but we didn't buy it. Medicine wasn't about following directions in a textbook. That's *not* what we were supposed to do. What we were supposed to do was save people—and so often, it seemed, we didn't.

"You want the truth?" we'd ask ourselves ruthlessly. "Here's the truth: a young woman came to you alive, breathing, fear in her eyes, wanting you to save her, and now she's lying on a metal cart in the morgue with a sheet over her. There's your truth for you."

So we would drag ourselves into the surgical waiting room, to the frightened, anxious eyes that had been waiting for us for the last three hours. The same eyes that looked to us with pleading and hope as we rushed their daughter to the OR. They knew before we said a word. They could see it in our struggle to speak.

"I . . . I am so sorry to tell you that . . ."

And afterward we'd sit on the bench in the doctors' locker room, and take a deep breath and slowly let it out—but we couldn't exhale everything. We'd sit there, hands folded and heads bent, too lethargic to pull off our bloody scrubs, too tired to go to bed, too dispirited to start that IV the nurses had called for two hours ago; our minds slowly going out of focus, slowly retreating from the horrors of the past few hours.

And if we were one of the lucky ones, we'd go off duty at eight or nine, after morning rounds. We'd drive home through avenues of early-morning sunlight flashing at us through the trees, hurting our eyes, like looking into the revolving lights on an ambulance. We'd come home to our wives who needed us. We'd mumble our hellos, brush past them, and tumble into a dreamless sleep.

But more likely we did not have the day off. We had another full day

ahead of us. And we had no time to think about what we did the night before. If the patient was still alive, there were other, newer challenges ahead.
His lytes were off. His output was down. His wound was bleeding. These
things demanded our attention, and we gave it gladly rather than try to quiet
the ghosts of the night before, of all the nights before, of all the whirling
maelstrom of amputated limbs and shotgun blasts and pussed-out bellies
and corn-picker hands and wide-open ankle bones filthy with asphalt and
dirt.

We were learning that all the training and all the caring in the world
were not going to solve every problem. This wasn't medical school. We
weren't going to ace every exam. Silver-haired professors weren't going to
pat us on the head and marvel at our intellectual acumen. We weren't going
to win every battle.

"Sometimes there's just too much trauma," Joe said.

There certainly had been for me.

# CHAPTER EIGHT

*November*

On a blustery Saturday morning, with three inches of new snow on the ground, I sat in the ER of St. Mary's Hospital for one last morning report. Jerry was still up in surgery where they had taken a guy with a ruptured bowel about 4:00 A.M. Mac was slumped in a chair in the corner. Rollie and I were relatively fresh, having had the night off. Joe Stradlack thanked us, said we did a good job, and then began to orient the new guys.

When morning report was over, Rollie, Mac, and I shook hands. They said for a dumb orthopod I did all right. I thanked them and wished them good luck taking care of rectal abscesses and fat people's gallbladders for the rest of their lives.

I asked them to say good-bye to Jerry for me, and I headed to the docs' lounge to begin my next assignment: six weeks in pediatric orthopedics. Jake Burg, my new senior resident, knew I had just come off the ERSS. I think he felt sorry for me. After we finished rounds he told me to take the rest of the weekend off.

Jack Manning, who had started on Dr. Hale's service that morning, gave me a ride to Methodist Hospital for the Saturday morning conference. On ERSS we were never given time off for conferences, so I hadn't been to one since September. The conference was on complications of carpal navicular fractures. I was just settling into my chair when Dr. Burke called on me.

"Dr. Collins, how nice of you to join us. Explain the high incidence of nonunion and osteonecrosis associated with navicular fractures."

I explained that navicular fractures were often accompanied by disruption of the vascular supply to a portion of the bone.

"Which portion of the bone?"

"The distal portion."

"What is the name of the vessel that is disrupted?"

"I believe it's a branch of the—"

"You believe?"

"It's a branch of the radial artery. It enters the navicular at the—"

"I didn't ask you where it entered. I asked you the name of it."

"Tell him it's the anal artery," Frank Wales whispered from behind me.

"I'm sorry, Dr. Burke. I can't recall the name."

"Don't apologize to me," he answered. "It's your poor patient you should apologize to."

I mumbled, "Yes, sir," and started to sit back down.

"When was the last time you attended this conference, Dr. Collins?"

I stood back up. "It's been a few weeks, sir, but I've been—"

"I don't care where you've been. Attendance at this conference is mandatory."

"But I thought when we were on—"

"Mandatory."

I realized I should cut my losses and shut up. "Yes, sir," I said.

"Mandatory, that is, for those who wish to remain in this residency program."

"Yes, sir."

I stood in silence while he stared at me from over the top of his reading glasses. "Sit down, Dr. Collins," he said finally. "Dr. Manning, do you know the name of the vessel that supplies the navicular?"

As I plopped back in my chair, Frank touched me on the shoulder. "I think he likes you," he whispered.

By 11:30 I was home. Although he lived on the opposite side of town, Jack had given me a ride.

"Look what I found, Patti," he called as we pulled into the driveway. "He doesn't look like much but he's housebroken—sort of."

The sun had come out and last night's snow was already starting to melt. Patti was standing at the curb, next to our car, an old green Dodge that hadn't started in four days. She was wearing a cream-colored, Irish cardigan sweater that fell to either side of her very swollen belly. Eileen stood next to her, both hands wrapped around Patti's right leg. Mr. Jensen from the Standard station was there, too. He looked up, nodded in my direction, and then stuck his head back under the hood.

Jack told Patti she was looking good. "I like that beach ball look," he said.

"Ha-ha, very funny," she said, sticking out her tongue at him.

Jack backed out of the driveway, waved, and said to call him if we needed a ride anywhere. When he was gone, I went over to Pat and gave her a kiss. She looked worried.

Mr. Jensen straightened up and slammed the hood. "Mornin', Doc," he said.

"Hi, Mr. Jensen. So, what do you think?" I asked, pointing at our car.

He didn't waste any time. "Engine's blown," he said. "Cost you two grand, maybe more, to fix it."

Two grand? We only paid seven hundred for it.

Jensen saw the look on my face. "Forget it. It ain't worth fixin'."

Patti and I stood there saying nothing.

"Sorry, Doc," Jensen said. As he was getting into his truck, he turned to me and said, "I gave Mrs. C. the number of a guy I know owns a junk-yard. He might give you thirty or forty bucks for it."

I smiled weakly. I wondered if he was trying to be funny. When he left, Patti and I turned to each other.

"Now what?" she said.

"How much money do you have?" I asked.

She dug in her pockets. "Six dollars."

I put my arm around her. "We've got three hundred in the bank, plus whatever we get from the junkyard . . ."

She looked at me. "Do you really think we'll only get thirty dollars for it?"

Ten minutes later I was on the phone to Ernie Hausfeld, owner of the Mantorville Junkyard.

"Collins? Oh, yeah. Old man Jensen said you might call. He says you're a doctor at the Mayo, huh?"

"Yes, that's right."

"Then how come you're driving a junker?"

Oh, yeah, I forgot. Doctors always drive Porsches and BMWs. "My Lamborghini's in the shop," I told him, "so I've been driving my butler's car. I thought I'd get him a new one."

"Very funny, Doc. Well, here's the deal: if you can drive the car here, I'll give you thirty-five dollars for it. If we have to tow it in, you get twenty-five."

Twenty-five dollars, that's it?

I sighed. "The engine's blown, Ernie. You'll have to come and get it."

"All right. Have the title ready. Someone'll be there in an hour."

Three hours later a tow truck pulled up in front of the house. A young guy with a dirty blue Twins cap got out and looked at our address. I walked out to meet him. He glanced at the paper in his right hand. "Doc Connolly?" he asked.

"Collins," I said, holding out my hand.

He stuck the paper back in his pocket and shook hands with me. "I'm Jimmy. I drive for Ernie." He looked at the Dodge. "This your car?"

I nodded. "Yup. That's it."

"So the old girl's headed for the last roundup, huh?"

"Yeah. I hate to see her go. She always ran great—until the last few days."

"You got anything in the trunk or glove compartment?"

"Nope." The spare tire was bald but it held air, so I had rolled it into the garage on the odd chance that it would fit whatever "new" car we got.

Jimmy backed up the tow truck, and hooked the winch under the front bumper. He pressed a button on the side of his truck, and the front of the car rose off the ground.

"I just need the title," he said, "and we're all set."

I handed it to him. He, in turn, counted out five dirty five-dollar bills and gave them to me.

"Pleasure doing business with you, Doc."

Patti came out and watched as Jimmy drove away with our car.

"Want to come down to the BMW dealership with me to pick out our new Beemer?" I asked.

She wasn't laughing. "Mike, what are we going to do?"

"I looked at some ads in the *Post-Bulletin*. I think we can get something decent for six or seven hundred dollars."

"Where are we going to get six or seven hundred dollars?"

"I thought I'd get a job as a male stripper."

"Yuk." She grimaced. "Who would hire you? Nursing homes for blind, senile old ladies?"

If you want to stay grounded, get married. Still, there was no need to rub it in.

I told Patti I didn't have a plan. I said we'd just have to wait for our next paycheck, which was two weeks away.

"How much money do we need?"

"Well, three, four hundred bucks, I guess. Plus the three hundred we have in the bank."

I turned and started walking back toward the house, but Patti stood where she was.

"Aren't you forgetting something?" she asked.

"Like . . .?"

"Like there won't be any money left for food."

"I'll bring stuff home from the hospital when I'm on call."

"I'm not living on apples and prune sweet rolls for a month," she said.

"If you treat me right I just might bring home a little lutefisk casserole."

She grabbed Eileen's hand and stormed by me.

"I don't want lutefisk casserole," she said. "I want meat. And vegetables. And potatoes."

"Damned Irish girls," I called after her. "I should have married an Indian woman. She could have lived off roots and berries and grubs for a month."

"And I should have married a lawyer. At least there'd be food on the table."

Patti had been under a lot of stress or she never would have said such a terrible thing.

# CHAPTER NINE

*November*

As autumn drew to a close we were starting to settle in. I was enjoying my stint on pediatric orthopedics. Patti, meanwhile, had met all the neighbors. She was a regular customer at Mr. Jensen's Standard station. She had made friends with Dan the Butcher at Barlow's grocery store, and Tim the Mailman, and Zack the Garbageman. I was constantly running into people who said, "You must be Patti's husband."

We had gotten a new car, a '72 Pontiac I bought from a guy out near the airport. It had no shocks, the brakes squeaked, and it was badly rusted, but it started easily enough. For six hundred dollars I wasn't going to get anything better.

"Why does the front seat wobble like that?" Patti asked when she first got in.

I had forgotten to tell her the bolts for the front seat had rusted out.

"It's so you can rock the babies while I'm driving," I said.

She gave me one of her looks. "Did you have to pay extra for it?"

"Aw, come on, hon. What did you think we were going to get for six hundred bucks?"

She relented a little. "Well, the tires don't look so bad. But are you sure it's safe to drive Eileen in this thing?"

"Unless she can find a better set of parents, she's stuck with us—and our car."

I was getting more comfortable with orthopedics. I still felt behind all the other residents, but at least I was learning the language. Now that I was off ERSS, call was a little more tolerable. I was on call every third or fourth night. When I was on call I had to stay in the hospital, and was responsible for taking care of orthopedic problems in the ER, seeing consults, and answering pages from the nurses on the ortho floor. I would rarely sleep for more than two or three hours. But at least I was home with Patti and Eileen most nights.

Eileen had always slept in a crib next to Patti, but with another baby on the way we thought Eileen should get used to her own room. We decided to turn one of our other rooms into a nursery.

But moving Eileen into a room by herself seemed so cruel, so selfish. What if she choked? What if she got tangled up in the blankets and cut off the circulation to her legs? What if she chewed through an electrical cord while her rotten parents were in the other room enjoying themselves? What then, huh?

But she was sixteen months old; she slept all night anyway, so why would she care? The problem, of course, was not *her* ability to accept the change. It was ours. The first night we moved Eileen to her new room, Patti got up three times to make sure she was okay.

"Did you hear that?" Patti asked sometime in the middle of the night.

"Huh?" I said, jerking awake. It was still dark out.

"I thought I heard Eileen."

I sighed and rolled over.

"Mike!" She shook my shoulder. "It's Eileen. I think she's fussing."

"She is not. It's just that greasy-looking guy with the ax I saw in there before we went to bed."

"I hate you," she said, yanking the covers off me and getting up to check our daughter.

"That's not what you said a couple hours ago," I said as she stormed from the room.

She flopped back in bed two minutes later and stuck a cold foot in the middle of my back.

"Some father you are."

"Mrrmph."

A week later I came across a small notice in the *Fellows Newsletter*. The Mayo Clinic Fellows Hockey Team was starting its new season. All interested players were invited to attend the first practice at 8:00 A.M. Sunday, November 26, at Graham Arena. I was thrilled. Here, at last, was something I could do. Orthopedically I was still the lowest of the low, the guy who knew less than everyone about everything. But hockey was different. Hockey was my game. I had played for Notre Dame—not that I was a star, but I was good enough to letter for two years. I was a fringe player in college, having made it more on desire than on talent. My only claim to fame was that I briefly held three all-time records at Notre Dame: Most Penalties in a Game, Most Penalties in a Season, and Most Penalties in a Career.

Although I hadn't played much since graduation, I was confident I had the ability to play with anyone. I was anxious to get on the ice again and was delighted to learn the fellows had a team.

I didn't look like much that first Sunday morning. The only decent equipment I had were the skates, gloves, and shin guards I took with me when I graduated from Notre Dame. The rest of my equipment was a ragtag collection of outdated junk from high school. My jersey was a flea-bitten rag with *O'Dea's Pub* stenciled across the front.

I was leaning over, lacing my skates, when someone stepped in front of me.

"*You* play hockey?"

I looked up to see Dr. Jonathan Wilhelm sneering at me. Ever since that breakfast when I was on Harding's service, Wilhelm never missed an opportunity to ridicule me. I was the butt of all his jokes. Every morning he would make some comment about "the world's dumbest resident," and would wonder how long it would be until I was kicked out of the program.

Wilhelm was from Edina, a wealthy suburb of Minneapolis. When he wasn't talking about what a wonderful surgeon he was, he was bragging about what a great hockey player he had been in high school.

He stood over me. "Where are you from, Collins?"

"Chicago."

"Chicago? Chi-CAW-go?" He started laughing and then called to several other residents, none of whom I knew. "Hey, we've got Bobby Hull here. He's from Chicago."

Wilhelm slipped on his helmet, being careful not to mess his hair. He then tapped me nonchalantly on the head with his stick. It was a tap, but it hurt. "Nice jersey, Bobby," he said.

There were a few snickers. But I also noted there were several players who said nothing. Presumably they had spent some time in proctology and recognized an asshole when they saw one. Wilhelm laughed again and strode out of the locker room.

The top of my head was a little sore, but I couldn't have been happier. Wilhelm was a hockey player! It was almost too good to be true. They say anticipation has its own rewards. Until that moment, however, I had never fully experienced the truth of that adage. I savored what was going to happen next.

Suddenly I was in no hurry. I checked my blades, running a thumbnail across each edge. I laced and relaced my skates. I carefully wrapped a roll of 1 ½" tape around my shin guards. Not a damn thing had happened, but I was already enjoying myself more than I had in months. The locker room slowly emptied as the other players dressed and went on the ice. When the last player left the locker room, I sat there alone. I could hear the Zamboni come off the ice, and then the report of slap shots and the boom of pucks hitting the boards.

But still I waited. I wanted to be the last guy on the ice, the guy with the shitty equipment who would be the last one picked for the scrimmage. The only thing I cared about was being sure I wasn't on Wilhelm's team—but I figured Wilhelm would see to that.

Finally, as the sound of the slap shots died down, I knew they were picking teams. I did a few stretches to loosen up, then I took out my front teeth and dropped them in the pocket of my pants. This was going to be a hell of a morning.

"You should be ashamed of yourself," Patti said that night after I told her the story. "You're practically thirty years old—"

"I'm nowhere near—"

"You're practically thirty years old," she continued, "you're married, you have a little baby and another one on the way. You're supposed to be a doctor, and you go around acting like some kind of a stupid barroom brawler."

"Actually, the correct term, in hockey circles, is not 'stupid barroom brawler.' It's 'goon.' I was acting like some kind of a goon."

"Go ahead and make jokes, but what if this Wilhelm person makes trouble for you?"

"You mean what if he tells his mommy?"

"No, Mike, what if he tries to make you look bad at conferences or if he starts telling attendings about you?"

"About how stupid I am?"

"That's not what I meant."

"Yes, it is. But it's okay. You don't have to worry. Today Dr. Wilhelm and I came to an understanding. Although I chose not to appeal to his rational side, I still managed to be rather persuasive. I'm sure he will henceforth see our relationship in a new light."

And he did. The next morning at breakfast I placed my tray on the table and sat down right next to him. I never looked at him, never said a word to him. I just ate my breakfast. But, for the first time, Dr. Wilhelm, who seemed to be having some difficulty chewing, had nothing to say to or about me, either.

# CHAPTER TEN

*December*

I liked pediatric orthopedics. After the unrelenting intensity of the ERSS, it was nice to deal with mundane kids' problems for a while. But peds ortho wasn't all flat feet and pigeon toeing. This was the Mayo Clinic and we got our share of difficult cases, too.

Bobby Lang was a six-year-old kid transferred to us from Decorah, Iowa. He had ridden his bike down a hill, directly into the path of a bread truck. He was lucky, though. Except for a laceration on the back of his head, his injuries were confined to the left leg. He had fractured his femur, and had torn away much of the skin on the front of his lower leg. The guys on ERSS made sure there were no other injuries, stitched up the back of his head, and then turned Bobby over to us.

Jake Burg was the senior resident on Peds with me. We got a big basin and several thousand cc's of antibiotic solution and spent over an hour irrigating and picking pieces of dirt and asphalt from Bobby's leg. It was obvious he would eventually need skin grafting. While I finished dressing the wounds, Jake took the X-rays upstairs to Dr. Steinburg, our attending surgeon. When Jake got back I asked him how Steinburg wanted to treat the femur fracture.

"Ninety-ninety traction," Jake replied. That meant Bobby would not have surgery, but would be put in traction for four to six weeks, lying on his back with both his hip and his knee bent to ninety degrees.

Traction is applied to a fractured leg by drilling a pin through the bone distal to the fracture site. Weights are then attached to the pin to pull the bone back into alignment.

When I told Jake I had never put in a femoral traction pin, he said it was time I learned. He asked the nurses to get a skeletal traction tray and then showed me the landmarks I would use to put in the pin.

"All right," Jake said when the tray arrived. "Let's do it."

I looked at him in amazement. "Right here?" I said. "Aren't we going to bring him to the OR and do it under general anesthesia?"

"Nope. We're doing it right here, in the bed."

Traction pins are put in with a hand drill. I knew that much. A small puncture wound is made in the skin. Then a threaded pin is poked through the hole, pushed up against the cortex of the bone, then drilled through and out the other side. I had never seen it done but I knew it must be incredibly painful. And we were going to do this to a six-year-old boy *without anesthesia*? He couldn't be serious.

"Mike," Jake told me, "it's not that big a deal. We do it all the time. You don't put someone under general anesthesia for a simple procedure that takes two minutes. The kid is already in a ton of pain. We'll give him a shot of morphine, put the pin in, hang him up in traction, and within a day or two he'll be feeling a hell of a lot better."

That was well and good, but he sure wouldn't be feeling "a hell of a lot better" when I drilled an eighth-inch Steinmann pin through his femur.

It reminded me of doing circumcisions. When I was on my OB rotation in med school the residents had let me do all the "circs." At first I was thrilled, but I grew to hate it. There was no anesthesia, nothing. We just took the poor baby's foreskin, stretched it out, and chopped it off. "Wiener whacking," the residents called it. The poor baby would scream his guts out. The OB residents seemed not to mind. They were inured to it. Even the most compassionate of them would look at the screaming infant, shrug his shoulders, and say, "Poor little guy. Well, get used to it, junior. Life's a bitch." I think they had convinced themselves that little babies were like carrots: if they couldn't articulate their pain, they must not have any.


Jake told Bobby's parents we had to put a pin in his leg. He asked them to step out for a few minutes. When they were gone he put a blanket under Bobby's knee to keep it bent. Despite the morphine, Bobby howled in pain. When Jake had the leg in the correct position he helped me prep the end of the femur.

"Couple things," Jake said as he loaded the Steinmann pin into the chuck. "First of all, stay away from the growth plate. If you drill a traction pin through the growth plate his leg'll wind up three inches shorter than the other one."

I swallowed and nodded weakly.

"Second thing. Put the pin through the middle of the bone, okay? The exact middle. Walk the point of the pin up and down the cortex to be sure you are starting right in the middle. Then just crank the handle until the point of the pin goes through the bone and starts poking into the skin on the other side. Then I'll make a small incision so it can poke through. Got it?"

I nodded again.

"All right, Doctor. Let's go."

I pulled on my sterile gloves and picked up the hand drill. Jake took an 11-blade scalpel and made a small puncture wound on the inside of the distal thigh. "There's your starting point," he said.

At the head of the bed, Bobby was whimpering and moaning. Trying to look like I had done this before, I approached the side of the bed and smiled reassuringly at Bobby. As I moved the drill toward his leg, Bobby began to tremble. Tears poured from his wide eyes. Fortunately, because of the fracture, he couldn't move his leg. I brought the drill closer, the point hovering just outside the puncture wound Jake had made.

"Hold it," Jake said. "You have to angle it more *that* way." He pushed my elbow down a little. "Yeah, like that."

Slowly I advanced the pin through Bobby's muscle until I felt the tip of the drill jar against the femur.

"Now walk it up and down until you feel both the anterior and the posterior cortex," Jake said. As I did, Bobby's shaking sobs intensified.

"Okay?" Jake asked.

"Yeah," I said. "I'm right in the middle."

"All right, then drive it through."

As I slowly turned the handle, the threaded pin began burrowing into the femur. I glanced at Bobby who was groaning and tossing his head back and forth. I kept turning the handle until I could feel the pin exit the bone. A few more cranks and I could see the pin begin to tent the skin on the opposite side.

"Good," Jake said. "Now wait 'til I make an incision." He picked up the scalpel and made another short incision. Bobby scarcely said a thing this time. After having someone drill a pin through his bone, a little stab wound didn't seem to faze him.

Another twenty seconds and I had the pin centered through the thigh, about three inches sticking out on each side.

"I *like* it!" Jake said. "Now let's slip on the traction bow, and hook up the weights."

Fifteen minutes later we had the X-rays back. "Good job," Jake said. "See how you're a couple inches above the growth plate? That's perfect. Now we have to get the leg lined up."

We set up a series of pulleys to allow Bobby's femur to be pulled straight up toward the ceiling. His knee was bent to ninety degrees, parallel to the bed, resting on a cloth sling. A series of weights dangled from the traction bar at the foot of the bed. This whole process must have been incredibly painful to Bobby, but by then he was so washed out, so despairing of our ever being done, that he just moaned constantly no matter what we did.

Finally, when it was all over, we dressed the pin sites and let Bobby's parents come back in. When his mother bent over to kiss Bobby, his sobs intensified and he clung to her neck as though he would never let go.

But Bobby's torment wasn't over. Because of the damage to the skin on his lower leg, we had to change his dressings every day. Invariably the dressings would be stuck to the wound and no matter how gentle we tried to be, it was sheer torture to Bobby. Finally, one morning we took him to the operating room and took a skin graft from the front of his right thigh and applied it to the damaged area on his left leg.

I dreaded our visits to Bobby's room even more than he did. If an adult had this injury it wouldn't be so bad. He would understand that everything we did was for his own good. He *had* to have a pin drilled through his femur. He *had* to have dressings changed. He wouldn't have liked it, but he would have understood the necessity of it.

Bobby understood nothing. All he knew was that big men came to his room every day to hurt him. They strapped him down, and drilled pins through his bones. They twisted his broken leg. They ripped the skin off one leg, and tore at the sores on the other.

For the month we had Bobby in the hospital I watched the look in his eyes change from anxiety to fear, to hatred, and finally, worst of all, to despair. Toward the end of the month he no longer whimpered when we came in the room. He just lay there staring at us out of empty, sunken eyes, never flinching as we did our work.

A month later, when Bobby's skin graft had taken and his femur had started to heal, it was time to take him out of traction, put him in a cast, and let him go home. But first the traction pin had to be removed. Jake offered to let me do it, but I said no. I couldn't bear to have that little boy's eyes on me anymore.

"Jake," I said, "I just can't . . ." Jake looked at me strangely, shrugged, and said okay, he'd do it.

We slowly unhooked the traction and removed the traction bow from the pin. Then Jake got a big pin-cutter and cut one side of the pin flush with the skin. He attached the hand drill to the other side and backed the pin out. There was no crying or thrashing this time, just those haunted eyes staring out of the vacuum of his soul. It was unnerving, and it was Bobby's revenge. You hurt me, those eyes said. Now remember what you did to a little child, and remember what these eyes have to tell you about the human condition.

There was knowledge in those eyes, knowledge no child should ever have to possess, knowledge no adult ever *wants* to possess.

We put Bobby in a cast and let him go home the next day. Everything was healing nicely. His femur was straight. His skin had healed. I hoped someday he would thank us. But the straight femur and the healed skin had come at a great cost. I wondered how long it would take the rest of Bobby to heal. I wondered if he would ever again be able to look at the world through the eyes of a little boy.

I spent a lot of time thinking about Bobby after he had gone, trying to analyze my feelings. I was gratified that things had turned out so well, but I also felt guilty about all the pain we had inflicted on him. I concluded that it was naive to think all Bobby's problems could be completely and instantly and painlessly cured. We weren't gods, we were just a bunch of guys trying to do the best we could for injured people. We did what we could to help Bobby. *We* didn't break his femur, we mended it. *We* didn't rip the skin off his leg, we grafted it. Yes, what we did was painful, but it was necessary. That boy would have been crippled for life if we hadn't helped him.

I had changed a lot over the previous six months. I had learned to keep my emotions a little more in check. I was a little more hardened, a little more seasoned, but the suffering of a little boy still got to me. And yet I knew if I wanted to be a surgeon I was going to have to get used to some harsh realities. Mothers die. Kids get run over by trucks. And sometimes the things we do to help them cause pain. Yes, I needed to be compassionate, but I couldn't let my compassion paralyze me. I had to believe in what I was doing. I had to believe in the essence of a surgeon's art: that a scalpel can heal every bit as much as it can cut.

# CHAPTER ELEVEN

*December*

"Don't you ever return phone calls?" my brother Denny asked. "This is the third time I've called you."

I told him I was sorry and mumbled something about never being home.

"Yeah, well listen," he said. "My right shoulder's been bothering me, and it's getting worse. I know you're only a resident but I thought maybe you could tell me what's the matter."

I didn't like the "only a resident" crack. "Shoulder? What's a shoulder? Hold on. Let me look it up in my medical dictionary."

"Come on. I mean it. The damn thing's been killing me after hockey and now it's even keeping me up at night."

"Have you tried warm milk and a pacifier?"

"Hey, dickhead, are you going to help me or not?"

"All right. Go ahead."

He told me he had injured his shoulder playing football in college, and that "the damn thing has never been right since." He had some free time next week and would come up to Mayo if I could get an appointment for him.

"But I don't want to see some resident," he said. "Make sure you line me up with someone good."

Oh, so we're back to insulting residents again, huh? Okay. "I know the perfect guy for you," I said. "He just got his license reinstated. He finished rehab and is living in a halfway house with his old lady who is sixteen. He hardly ever uses acid when he operates now. And you'll love his tattoos— but at least he's not a resident."

This wasn't the best time for us to be having visitors. Patti had just given birth to our second daughter, Mary Kate. The delivery went smoothly, but Pat was tired and sore. I tried to get her to look at things philosophically.

"Look," I said. "Nature, in her infinite wisdom, has decreed the manner by which babies are brought into this world. I did my part willingly and cheerfully. I think you should do the same."

She mentioned something about "willingly and cheerfully" performing an operation with a rusty knife that would allow me to sing in the Vienna Boys Choir.


Four days later, Denny arrived in his beat-up Jeep. He tossed his suitcase on our bed. "This'll be fine," he said, "but where are you and Patti going to sleep?"

"Get that roach-infested thing off our bed," I said, kicking his suitcase onto the floor. "You're going to the basement."

The two of us went down to the basement where we cursed and kicked open the couch-bed. Denny pushed on the musty lump of petrochemicals we had just unfolded into his mattress. "The hell with my shoulder," he said. "I'm gonna need a spine fusion by the time I get out of this place."

"No, please," I said, holding up a hand. "Don't thank me. Just seeing that look of brotherly affection in your eyes is all the thanks I'll ever need."

He gave me the finger and yelled up the stairs, "Patti! Why did you ever marry this loser?"

I didn't see Denny again for four days. I was on call the day after he arrived. The following night I came home at six and went to bed at seven. On the third night I was on call again.

When I came home on the fourth day, Denny was sitting at the kitchen table holding Mary Kate on his lap and drinking a beer. He had seen

Mayo's shoulder guru, had an X-ray and an MRI scan, and was scheduled for surgery in the morning.

Patti had told me how great it was having him around—"since you never are," she said. In between clinic appointments, Denny fed Eileen, helped with the shopping, shoveled the sidewalk, fixed the kitchen faucet, and generally did everything a real husband would do. And now he was sitting with my infant daughter on his lap. She sat there contentedly chewing on her knuckle and drooling all over the front of his shirt.

"Want a beer?" Denny asked. He was very generous with my beer.

I opened the refrigerator. I had purchased a case of Grain Belt the week before. There was one left. I popped the top of the last beer and sat back down. "What happened to the rest of the case?" I asked.

He leaned forward and lowered his voice. "Patti," he whispered, nodding slightly toward the sink. "I think you may have a little problem on your hands there." He made a drinking gesture with the thumb of his right hand.

"Has she been pouring them on her Cheerios again?" I asked.

He shrugged his shoulders. "It's tragic, simply tragic. God knows I've tried to help." He looked at Mary Kate playing on his lap, and shook his head. "My heart goes out to these poor children."

"What are you two whispering about over there?" Patti asked. She turned off the faucet and wiped her hands on the front of her apron. She came over, put her hands on my shoulders, and kissed the top of my head.

"Your boozehound brother-in-law is trying to bullshit his way out of responsibility for the fact that we are out of beer."

"Out of beer?" She opened the refrigerator and stared incredulously. "Out of beer?"

I turned to Denny and flashed a smug smile. Now he was in for it.

Pat swung the door shut and turned on me. Me! "How could you?" she said. "The only job I gave you was to make sure we had enough beer for your brother. I can't believe you ran out."

*I* ran out? I, the guy who had been working almost four days in a row? I, the guy who barely had one sip of one beer? I ran out?

I turned and looked at Denny who was gazing innocently out the window, the same faint, shit-eating grin on his face as when he used to get me in trouble with Mom. I looked back at Patti who was standing with her hands on her hips, glaring at me.

Okay.

I stood up, belched loudly, and began swaying back and forth, beer in my right hand. "All right, I ran outta beer. Whassa matter? Can't a guy have a coupla beersh around here?"

Patti rolled her eyes. "Knock it off and go to Barlow's and get some more beer for your brother."

"C'mere, baby," I said, staggering forward. "I'm just a lonely truck-drivin' man." I groped for her and started singing, *"Six days on the road and I'm a-gonna make it home tonight."*

She laughed, pushed me away, and looked over my shoulder at Denny. "Take this lunatic to the store and have him get you some more beer."

We got the beer and returned home to a chicken and mashed potatoes dinner (Denny's favorite). I asked why we never had *my* favorite dinner, pot roast, and was promptly told to shut up, that I wasn't the one having surgery the next day, and besides, I didn't exactly look like I was starving to death. That was a low blow. I was going to start working out again as soon as things slowed down a little.

Since it was the night before his surgery, Denny had been told not to drink alcohol, so he said he would have only four more beers—which was just as well. It was 8:30 and I couldn't keep my eyes open.

His surgery went well. They kept him in the hospital overnight and sent him home the following morning. Patti talked him into staying in town for a week until they took his stitches out. Even with his right arm in a sling he was still able to rock the baby and play with Eileen.

I didn't see much of Denny after surgery. I was on call a lot, and even when I was home I didn't have much gas left in the tank. I would drag myself in the back door, halfheartedly pick at dinner, and then drop into bed.

Four days after Denny's surgery I got home about 6:00 P.M. Denny was in the living room rocking the baby. She was sleeping peacefully on his shoulder.

"Let me hold that sweet little thing," I said to him. I reached over and lifted Mary Kate from his shoulder. She immediately started fussing and squirming.

"Not like that," Denny said. "She doesn't like to be held that way."

I shifted her around but she continued to cry.

"Never mind," he said. "Just give her back to me. She doesn't like strangers."

I was her father. I wasn't a stranger. Nevertheless, stunned and crushed, I handed her back to Denny. He laid her on his shoulder, and patted her on the back. She snuggled a time or two, gave a contented sigh, and was still.

"Did Mister Stranger-Danger try to hurt you?" he cooed. "Don't worry. Uncle Denny won't let that bad man hold you again."

His teasing hit too close to home. What the hell kind of life am I leading? I wondered. I hardly ever see my wife. My kids don't even know me. My brother is more of a father to them, and more of a husband to Patti than I am. Is this what I want?

I felt frustrated and guilty—for about two minutes. An hour later Patti woke me up and said I should just go to bed. I wasn't any use to anyone passed out on the couch drooling all over the front of my shirt. I staggered to my feet. My guilt was forgotten. Everything was forgotten. I hung my pants on the top of the bathroom door, dropped my shirt on the floor, and fell into bed.

Denny left three days later. I never got to say good-bye. For weeks afterward Eileen would look at me when I walked in the back door, frown, and ask when Uncle Denny was coming home.

# CHAPTER TWELVE

*January*

On January 3 I started on Antonio Romero's service—one of the busiest services at Mayo. On my first night on call I managed only one hour's sleep. I came home tired and hungry—and it was snowing again, five inches on Sunday, three inches on Tuesday, six inches so far today, and three more on the way.

Why, I wondered, did the Mayo Brothers have to start their clinic in Minnesota? Hadn't they ever heard of Hawaii? At this very moment some guy is doing an ortho residency in Honolulu. He is running a clinic for surfing injuries. A voluptuous young thing approaches. "Doctor," she says, with a little pout, "I'm getting chafing from my halter top. Can you help me?"

Back in Minnesota, though, it was fifteen degrees and dumping—but at least I was prepared. I had made two extravagant purchases with my first paycheck in August. The first was a pair of Sorrel boots from the local Feed and Seed Store. Sorrel is the Canadian manufacturer of a legendary rubber-soled, felt-lined boot made to withstand the most extreme winter conditions. Minnesota ice fishermen swear by them. No matter how drunk they get, no matter how many other body parts become frozen stiff, their feet stay warm.

My second purchase had been a heavy, goose-down coat from L.L. Bean. The coat was a drab tan color with a dark brown corduroy collar and a detachable hood. It was supposed to keep you warm "in any kind of weather." So far it had.

It was only five o'clock but already it was pitch-black outside. Snow swirled around the light over the back door. I hated to leave the warmth of the kitchen, but if I didn't shovel the driveway I wouldn't be able to get out in the morning. I laced up the Sorrels, then zipped and buttoned my coat. I slipped out the back door and clumped through the drifting snow to the garage where I kept the heavy, cast-iron coal shovel I had inherited from some long-forgotten construction job.

I pulled down the garage door, then turned to face 140 feet of driveway that stretched to the street. I picked up the shovel. The sooner I started the sooner I'd be back inside where it was warm.

Back in Hawaii, my counterpart was treating his second patient: a college girl with second-degree sunburn from her first visit to the nude beach. "Hold all calls, Nurse," he said from behind the curtain. "This may take a while."

But in Minnesota there were no nude beaches, just snow-covered driveways. I started by shoveling a narrow swath down the middle of the driveway. Within five minutes I started to feel warm. I was wearing a wool hat so I pulled my hood back. The cold air on my neck felt good.

The shovel was indestructible. It could chop ice and drive through the most hard-packed snow. I literally made sparks fly with it. I stood at a right angle to the driveway, my feet wide apart as I drove the shovel into the snow. The shovel grated against the concrete, and I exhaled sharply as I hurled the snow to the side. I started to get into a rhythm, the numbing iamb of labor:

> Shhhk-*humpf!*
> Shhhk-*humpf!*
> Shovelin' snow
> Don't mean jack.
> Lord I want
> My baby back.
> Shhhk-*humpf!*
> Shhhk-*humpf!*

Every ten minutes I straightened up, leaned against the shovel, and stretched my back. I was sweating heavily. My coat was unzipped, and I had crammed my wool hat into one of the pockets. A layer of snow coated my hair as I shifted the shovel to my left hand. Another sixty feet to go.

In ninety minutes I was finished, but I looked with dismay where the drifting snow had already started to reaccumulate against the garage.

Back in Hawaii, the resident yawned. He had been working for almost three hours and he was exhausted. Sunset was still another four hours away. He wondered if he should have mahi or wahoo for dinner. He opted for the former. "The Vouvray is so much nicer with mahi, don't you think?" he asked Bambi.

Bambi was an exotic dancer who doubled as his cast technician. She giggled and said, "Oh, Doctor, I love it when you talk dirty."


The snow was bad, but the cold was worse. All through October and November blizzards and cold fronts gathered strength in the arctic reaches of northern Canada, biding their time until they swept across the frozen lakes and plains of Manitoba and the Dakotas to hurl themselves on us in a demented frenzy.

I awoke one Saturday to the coldest day I had ever seen. All night the wind had howled from the north, tearing a thin flume of snow from the drifts piled on either side of the road. Patti and I spent the night huddled next to each other under four covers.

Harley Flathers, the morning radio announcer on KROC, read a statement from the governor's office. "The National Weather Service has issued a severe weather warning for the entire state of Minnesota. Temperatures from minus twenty to minus forty with high winds are anticipated. Wind chills are estimated to be a hundred degrees below zero. The governor has declared a state of emergency and asks all citizens to remain indoors."

All over the city, cars wouldn't start or, worse, started only to die in the middle of nowhere. Water mains burst, deliveries ceased, gas pumps froze.

Mac Self, who had been on ERSS with me, was from Florida. I ran into him in the doctors' lounge as I was finishing rounds. Mac was not having a good day. He told me he had never seen cold like this. He felt like a damn Eskimo. He said a person had to be nuts to live in this godforsaken place.

"Why in the hell did I ever leave Ft. Myers?" he asked.

He told me the lock on his back door froze, the gas line in his car froze, the bottle of scotch in his trunk froze, the pipes in his basement froze, the cup of coffee on his dashboard froze, and his dog's penis froze.

"Listen to this." He was reading from the chapter on "Frostbite of the Extremities" in the ER Manual: "In the field, the initial treatment of severe frostbite is to warm the frozen digit by cupping it gently in your hands."

He dropped the book as if he had been stung. "I'll be goddamned," he said, "if I am going to take that dog's johnson in my hand. I don't care if it does fall off."

I was home by noon. Patti put the kids down for their nap and made a couple grilled cheese sandwiches for us. When we were done, she noticed I was pulling on my Sorrels. "Where do you think you're going?" she asked.

"I have to bring that chair back to Eamonn's," I said.

Eamonn O'Sullivan was an Irishman who had come to Mayo to do a fellowship in Neurology. The poor man had never seen a temperature below twenty degrees in his life. He was appalled when I called to say I would be right over with the chair we had borrowed.

"Are you daft, then?" he asked in his thick West Cork accent. "Have you not seen the weather outside? Sure, Jaysus, it's colder than bedamn."

"Hell, Eamonn, I'm only bringing over a chair. We're not going to play softball."

He begged me not to come, swore he didn't need the chair, said he would pick it up himself later in the week. "I don't want your death on me conscience," he said.

"I'll be there in fifteen minutes," I told him.

But first there was a car to start. The Ponch had started for me that morning, but only because I had gone out to start it during the night. I had become so attuned to its idiosyncrasies that I could tell almost instinctively how long to try, how long to rest between tries, how much to depress the accelerator, when to put it to the floor.

I bundled up in my L.L. Bean coat and went out to start the car. The garage door was frozen again so I backed up and threw a shoulder into it to break it loose. The two front doors of the car had been frozen shut for the last two days, so I had to get in through the back door and then climb over the front seat. The car coughed into life on the second try. I revved the engine a time or two and then left it running. I climbed out and sprinted back to the house to warm up. When I returned ten minutes later, the interior of the car had warmed up to about five below. I opened the trunk, tipped the chair into it, and set out for Eamonn's.

I headed up the hill next to the country club and then wound my way through the deserted streets to Eamonn's house. I left the car running, clambered over the seat, got out the back door, ran up to his apartment, and rang the bell. The wind was roaring out of the north, driving snow into my face, under my jacket, up my sleeves. I missed sitting in the car, not so much for the heat, but just to be out of the wind.

Eamonn opened the door, grabbed my arm, and yanked me in. He slammed the door behind me and began flapping his arms across his chest. "By God," he said, "it's colder than a Protestant's tit out there." Poor Eamonn and his wife, Moira, had shifted their baby, the TV, and a couple chairs into the kitchen—the only place in their basement apartment they could keep warm. The oven was on, the door open. Eamonn threw on several sweatshirts, two hats, and a coat and came out to help me carry the chair.

Afterward I sat in the kitchen with them having a cup of tea. While we watched a John Wayne movie I told them about Mac Self and his dog.

"The poor wee thing," Moira said.

We were silent for a while, watching the movie. Ten minutes later, after The Duke had whipped his man, I told them I'd better be going. I hoped my engine was still running.

I stood up and put my mug in the sink. The windows above the sink were frosted over. We could hear the wind howling. I pointed at the faucet. "You should leave the water running a trickle," I told Eamonn. "It keeps the pipes from freezing."

"It keeps the pipes from freezing," Eamonn repeated in wonder. He scratched some frost from the inside of the window, and then poured himself another mug of tea. "Lord Jaysus," he grumbled, cupping his hands around the warm mug. "It's a hundred degrees below zero, the wind is roarin' like the banshee, and we're huddled in the kitchen like a bunch of fuckin' refugees. Cars won't start, pipes are freezing, and dogs' dicks are falling off. What in the name of God sort of a place is this anyway?"

# CHAPTER THIRTEEN

*February*

I was still the junior resident on Dr. Romero's service when I met Susan Schenk. Susan was a forty-three-year-old kindergarten teacher from Winona, Minnesota, who came to our clinic one Monday morning complaining of left hip pain. The pain had started insidiously about a month earlier. A well-conditioned athlete who enjoyed her daily three-mile run, Susan had been forced to stop running because of the pain.

"Do you limp?" I asked.

She hesitated. "Well, my husband thinks I do."

"Do you have any pain at night?"

Susan nodded. "Yes," she said. "In fact, for the past week it's been waking me up almost every night. That's why I figured I'd better get over here and let you guys take a look."

I was becoming increasingly concerned. "Do you have any history of cancer?" I asked, trying to keep my voice casual.

"Nope, healthy as a horse," she answered.

"How about your parents or relatives—any cancer or anything there?"

"Well, my mother died of breast cancer a few years ago. But she was seventy-eight."

Susan said her general health was good. Yes, she'd been losing a little weight, but she attributed that to her running. She had also been feeling a little tired lately, but she said she wasn't concerned about that. "It's just this stupid hip," she said. "I'm sure it's nothing, but it won't go away."

Except for a little tenderness over the side of her hip, Susan's exam was normal. I sent her for a hip X-ray and went on to our next patient. Susan's X-rays were back two hours later. I stood outside her exam room, pulled the films out of the jacket, and held them up to the light. I winced and thought, Oh, no. Susan had a large lytic lesion in the subtrochanteric area of the femur.

I brought the films over to Dr. Romero. He stared at them for several seconds, then looked up at me. We both knew that the X-ray almost certainly indicated metastatic cancer, probably from the breast.

The two of us, somber-faced, went in to talk to Susan. Dr. Romero went through the same sort of history and physical as I had. He then told Susan the X-ray indicated a problem.

"Good!" she said with a laugh. "I was beginning to think it was all in my head."

When neither of us smiled, she must have sensed something was wrong.

"What is it?" she asked. "What's wrong? It's not arthritis, is it?"

"No, Mrs. Schenk, it's not arthritis."

There was another uncomfortable silence. Dr. Romero finally said, "We can't be sure at this point exactly what it is, but we need to run a few more tests."

Susan looked anxiously first at me, then at Dr. Romero, searching our faces for more information. She was starting to understand. "It's something bad, isn't it?"

Dr. Romero paused slightly and said, "It might be."

Her shoulders sagged, her head dropped on her chest, and she put her right hand over her eyes. "Oh, God," she whispered.

Dr. Romero took her hand and told her no definite diagnosis could be made yet. He said he was sorry to upset her, and sorrier still that it would be two days before the test results would be back. He offered to call her husband and talk to him.

Susan shook her head. "No," she said, "I'd rather not worry him."

I wrote out orders for a bone scan and several blood tests, then told Susan we would see her in two days to go over the test results with her. "In the meantime," I said, "you need to start using crutches. Your hip bone is weak and could break if you put too much pressure on it."

"It could break? Just from walking on it?" This was a woman who, just a few weeks ago, had been running three miles a day.

"Well, we don't want to take any chances," I told her.


Two days later while Susan and her husband were waiting in one of the exam rooms, Dr. Romero and I were down in radiology looking at the bone scan. Susan's entire skeleton was riddled with cancer. We could tell this wasn't primary bone cancer. It had spread from somewhere else.

"Could be thyroid or kidney," Dr. Romero said, "but the vast majority of cancers that present like this are from the breast."

I wondered how he was going to tell Susan and her husband. Long gone were the days when doctors would hide things like this from their patients. And yet we both wished there were some way we could spare them some of the terror and shock.

"I try to break it to them slowly," Dr. Romero said as we rode the elevator back to the fourteenth floor. "People can't process too much bad news all at once. They stop hearing what you say." He had obviously been through this many times before. He sighed and went on. "We already prepared Mrs. Schenk a little. She knows the tests might show a problem."

As we entered the exam room, Susan and her husband jumped to their feet and looked at us apprehensively. After brief introductions, Dr. Romero got right to the point. "I know you are anxious about the results of your tests," he began. "The bone scan confirmed that the spot we saw in your left hip appears to be a malignancy. That malignancy probably started somewhere else and spread, not only to your hip, but to a number of other bones as well."

With each pronouncement, Susan and her husband clung more desperately to each other. Relentlessly, Dr. Romero went on. "In addition, your blood tests indicate that you are anemic and that your liver may also be involved. All these things will have to be investigated."

The Schenks sat there in stunned silence for several seconds until Mr. Schenk said quietly, "What does all this mean?"

Although he would never have articulated his question this way, what he really meant was *Is my wife going to die?* And although we would never have articulated our response this way, the answer was *Yes.* I knew Dr. Romero wouldn't be that blunt. Not here. Not now. They needed a little time to absorb all this.

"It means your wife is a very sick woman," Dr. Romero said. "It means she is going to need a lot of help and a lot of treatment."

"So it's . . . cancer?" Susan asked.

"Yes, Mrs. Schenk, it's cancer."


We admitted Susan to the hospital that afternoon. A CT scan of her abdomen showed widespread metastatic disease. The oncologists examined her breast and found a large lump. Two days later, she had a radical mastectomy. Ten out of ten lymph nodes in her axilla were positive for cancer.

"Things are about as bad as they could be," the oncologist told us. "Even with chemotherapy and radiation I doubt she will live six months."

Things were happening so fast Susan could hardly take it all in. Within the space of three days she had gone from thinking she was a healthy woman with a sore hip to a condemned woman who was told she would be dead before the end of summer.

And to make matters worse, there was still the question of what to do about her hip.

"The cancer has eaten away some of the bone in your hip," Dr. Romero told her. "We can kill the cancer with radiation, but that will still leave a large, weak spot that could fracture."

"What can be done?" Susan asked.

"We could do what's called a prophylactic pinning. That means we wouldn't wait for the bone to break. We would go in now and put a plate and screws in to prevent the bone from breaking."

"Do you know for sure that it will break if I don't have the surgery?"

"No, Mrs. Schenk, we don't. But if we do nothing and the bone breaks, the surgery is much more difficult to perform."

Susan nodded and said nothing. She turned her head and looked out the window.

"Take some time to think about it," Dr. Romero said. "Talk to your husband. If you have any more questions you can talk to me or Dr. Collins anytime."

Later that afternoon, when I was making rounds by myself, Susan asked if she could talk to me about the operation. "What do you think I should do?" she asked.

The indications for surgery were clear: a one-inch lesion occupying greater than fifty percent of the diameter of the bone warrants prophylactic fixation. Period. The risk of fracture is too great otherwise. I explained that to her.

She nodded patiently. "Yes, but do *you* think I should have the operation?"

There was no doubt. The literature was clear. I started to say, "Of course, absolutely," but all that came out was, "I . . ."

Susan looked up at me from her bed, waiting for an answer. The answer should have been easy, but I hesitated. She had just undergone a radical mastectomy and an axillary node dissection. The general surgeons had opened her belly and closed it right back up when they found the disease was too widespread to operate on. She was constantly sick from the chemotherapy. And now we were proposing to do another major, painful operation for a problem that *might* occur?

"I doubt she will live six months," the oncologist had said.

Did we really need to add to her misery with another operation? The literature was clear, but the literature was only about *her femur.* Yes, it would be good for her femur to be prophylactically fixed, but that didn't mean it was good for Susan overall. Another operation meant more pain, more weakness, more debilitation. That was taking a lot from a woman with very little left to give.

But I was only a junior resident. Shouldn't I just stick to the party line and shut up?

"Susan," I said gently. "Do you realize that without the operation your hip may break, and if it does it will be a lot harder to fix than it is now?"

*"Please,"* she said. "I can't take any more of this. I don't want any more operations. I just want to go home."

I reached over and laid my hand on the top of hers. "So would I."


Susan declined the surgery and left the hospital two days later. For weeks I was terrified every time my beeper went off. I was afraid that it would be the ER calling to say Susan had fractured her hip. It would be all my fault. But the call never came.

Susan died at home on Easter Sunday. The day before she died, her hip broke as her sister rolled her over to change her sheets. Susan was in a coma by then and never knew it.

# CHAPTER FOURTEEN

*March*

As winter staggered into spring, and snow reluctantly gave way to sleet, we had just about run out of money. As a junior resident I took home $981.48 a month. It wasn't a lot for a guy with four mouths to feed—but, on the other hand, it was a hell of a lot more than I had made in medical school. I had three part-time jobs during my senior year in medical school: janitor, construction laborer, and dockman. I made enough money to keep a roof over our heads and buy a lot of meat loaf and potatoes. We weren't featured on *Life Styles of the Rich and Famous,* but we got by.

Patti and I had a lot of support when we lived in Chicago. Our parents had us over for dinner once a week. Her mother always sent us home with enough leftovers for at least one other meal. Any household items we needed some cousin or aunt already had: cribs, silverware, furniture, or baby clothes.

But when we moved to Rochester Patti and I were on our own. There were no free lunches (or dinners), no cousins showing up with old strollers, no aunts stopping by with some towels they "never used anyway," no uncles wanting to meet us at Horan's or Doc Ryan's for a burger and a beer.

As a resident I was now making twice as much, but we were spending twice as much as well. Bill Chapin did the math at breakfast one morning.

"We make about a grand a month at Mayo," he said. "That's two-fifty a week. We work about twelve hours a day on weekdays." He turned a napkin over and began jotting some figures. "Plus, say, four hours each on Saturday and Sunday. Now add to that one weekday and one weekend call, and that's another . . ." he thought for a moment, "maybe, thirty-two hours." He began totaling his numbers. "That means we work about a hundred hours a week. So, if I have done my math correctly, we are getting paid about $2.50 an hour."—

"We have to make sure this doesn't get out," Frank said. "If them dang lawyers find out how rich we are they'll swarm over us like flies on a cow pie."

It was funny in a way. We thought we should be paid more, but every one of us would have worked for nothing. We were being trained at the best place for orthopedic surgery in the world—and we knew it. We weren't just employees. We were students as well. The clinic owed us something for the work we did, but we owed them something for the education they gave us. All in all, $2.50 an hour seemed fair to both parties. They got cheap labor and we got a tremendous education. But, fair or not, I was having a hard time paying the bills on $2.50 an hour.

Patti and I were sitting at the kitchen table. I had just put the kids to bed. Patti had the paper spread in front of her. I was grumbling as I tried to balance the checkbook.

"How much do we have in our account?" Patti asked.

"Minus sixty dollars."

"Good thing I didn't marry you for your money."

"Well, it was for my body *and* my money, right?"

She made a funny sound in her throat, then asked, "How can our account have less than zero?"

"Because you keep spending money on frivolous things like food and clothes."

"Would you like your children to go around naked?"

"Well, no, not naked. That is, not the children . . ."

She gave me a look indicating she was not likely to be naked with me anytime in the next thirty years. I thought I'd better move on.

"Hon," I said, throwing down the pen and leaning back in my chair. "I think I'm going to have to start moonlighting."

"Moonlighting? How? Where?"

"I was talking to one of the senior residents, Steve Tucker. He said he could work me into the schedule at St. Joe's in Mankato a couple times a month."

A number of rural hospitals in southeastern Minnesota needed doctors to cover their emergency rooms—and they were willing to pay residents to do it. Immanuel St. Joseph's Hospital in Mankato, ninety miles west of Rochester, was one of them. Mayo residents had been staffing their ER for several years.

"Does the Clinic allow you to moonlight?" Patti asked.

"Not exactly."

" 'Not exactly?' That means no, doesn't it?"

"I'm not sure." I cleared my throat. "The Clinic . . . well, *discourages* moonlighting, but doesn't officially forbid it."

"So if BJ Burke catches you moonlighting will he say he's discouraged, or will he say you're fired?"

I shook my head. "I don't know. A lot of guys do it, but I don't know."

I knew some training programs completely outlawed moonlighting. Jack Manning told me his college roommate got kicked out of the general surgery program at Duke for moonlighting.

Steve Tucker said Mayo took a more sensible approach. "They know we don't moonlight so we can buy new Ferraris," he said. "We moonlight so we can buy food and pay mortgages. If you do your job and don't draw attention to your moonlighting, they'll let it slide. But if moonlighting starts interfering with the job you do as a resident, then they'll come down on you."

We had just gotten the kids to bed and were sitting on the couch in the living room listening to the Chieftains. Patti reluctantly agreed with my moonlighting plans, but wondered how often I would do it.

"Probably not more than a couple times a month," I told her. "And it's only on Friday, Saturday, or Sunday."

"So that means every weekend you're not on call at Mayo, you'll be moonlighting."

I hadn't thought of it that way. She was right. I was on call just about every other weekend at Mayo. The other two weekends per month I would now be in Mankato. I put my arm around her and she leaned against me. We sat there silent and miserable. This was going to be a disaster.

I called Steve Tucker the next morning and asked him to put me on the moonlighting rotation. I gave him a list of days I was available. I had to plan things carefully. Obviously I couldn't moonlight on a night I was already on call at Mayo. I also preferred not to moonlight the night before or the night after I was on call. One night without sleep was tolerable—two was courting disaster.

I also had to find someone to carry my beeper while I was away. Calls would come in. Problems would arise. Someone had to be available not only to answer questions, but also to go to the hospital if needed.

Bill, Frank, and Jack never hesitated when I asked them. They said they would cover for me anytime.


Three weeks later, on a Saturday morning, I was up at four. I finished rounds at Mayo and was on the road by 5:15. It was still dark as I headed west on Minnesota Highway 14 for my first day of moonlighting at St. Joe's Hospital in Mankato. Jack Manning had agreed to hold my beeper for me. ("But if you're not back by nine A.M. Sunday," he said, "I'm going to report you to BJ Burke.")

At 6:50 I pulled into the parking lot of Immanuel St. Joseph's Hospital. I went into the ER and saw three nurses sitting at the control desk. I asked if Dr. Leone was around. Jim Leone was the resident who had been moonlighting the night before. Steve Tucker had told me Leone would orient me to the place.

One of the nurses, a heavyset, fiftyish woman with frizzy brown hair, asked, "Are you Dr. Connolly?"

"No, Collins," I said.

"Dr. Collins?" She looked puzzled. "Dr. Leone said Dr. Connolly would be taking over."

"Where is Dr. Leone?"

"He just left. He said to tell you everything was fine. The place is empty except for the guy in four who sliced off the end of his tongue on a can of peaches."

I laid my shaving kit on the desk. "The end of his *what*?"

"Yeah, his tongue. Dr. Leone said it was a perfect case for your first day moonlighting."

I didn't like the look in her eyes.

"Hey!" came a voice behind one of the curtains in the corner of the room. "Izh shomebody gonna fish my fuckin' tongue or what?"

The nurse (*Connie* her name tag said) handed me a chart. "Mr. Berghof awaits you." She led me to the cart upon which a bearded man in a blood-stained Jerry Garcia T-shirt was sitting.

"Sit back down there, Al," she said, placing a hand on his chest and pushing him down. She turned to me. "Mr. Berghof got home from the tavern an hour ago. He opened a can of peaches with his pocketknife, pried back the lid, and was slurping down a peach when he cut his tongue on the edge of the lid."

"Fuckin' shing," Al muttered.

"Could I see your tongue, Mr. Berghof?" I asked.

" 'Ere uh izh," he said, sticking out his bloody tongue.

The tip wasn't completely severed. It was still dangling by a few strands of tissue. This would be interesting. I had never sewn a tongue back on.

I told Connie what instruments I would need. As she went to gather them, I considered how I would anesthetize the tongue. There was a nerve to the tongue—was it the glossopharyngeal or the hypoglossal? And which cranial nerve was that?

There are twelve cranial nerves: olfactory, optic, oculomotor, trochlear, trigeminal, abducens, facial, acoustic, glossopharyngeal, vagus, accessory, and hypoglossal. Medical students and nursing students always struggle to remember these nerves. Patti, in nursing school, had learned a pleasant little pneumonic that began: "On old Olympus's towering top" or something. We had learned a cruder version in medical school: "Ooh, ooh, ooh! To touch and feel a girl's vagina—ah, heaven."

All right, so what nerve was it—girl or heaven? I finally gave up and decided to do a local block.

"Mr. Berghof," I said, "I'm going to give you a shot near the base of the tongue to numb it up, okay?"

"Uh-huh," he said.

Connie, gloved, was pulling on Al's tongue, holding it between two gauze pads.

"All right," I said, holding up the syringe and squirting out the air, "now you hold real still while I give you the shot, okay?"

"Ahgle, ahgle," he said.

I nodded to Connie, indicating she should hold the tongue. Then I stuck the needle in the base of his tongue.

Al screamed and jerked his head away. He glared at me and said something that sounded very much like "You cogshugger."

"Mr. Berghof," I said, "you have to hold still."

Connie, who seemed to have little patience with drunks, grabbed his tongue again. "Did you hear what the doctor said, Al?" she asked, pulling on his tongue for emphasis. "He said to hold still."

Al's eyes bulged. "Aghaharble," he said and nodded his acquiescence.

I gave him three or four injections around the base of the tongue. Then I said we would wait a couple minutes for the anesthetic to take effect. It took me an hour, but I finally got the tip of his tongue sewn back on. I would have finished sooner but the smell of garlic chips and beer on his breath made me stop every couple minutes to turn my head and breathe.

"I think it's going to be okay, Mr. Berghof," I told him.

I snapped off my gloves and tossed them on the stand next to his cart. "You should stay away from solid foods for a few days. Stick with milk shakes, maybe a little custard, that sort of thing, okay?"

"Ah-kye."

As I turned to go he said, "Kedda habba kubba beerzh?"

I looked at Connie. "What did he say?"

Connie turned to him. "No, Al," she said, slapping him on the head with a towel. "You've had enough beers. Now go home and go to bed. And stay away from that can of peaches, too."

We were busy all day: lacerations, sprains, babies with ear pain, women with belly pain, men with chest pain. After my stint on the ERSS I was ready for just about anything. About 3:00 A.M. I finished treating a guy with a whiplash injury from a car crash. I sent him home with a cervical collar, a prescription for some pain meds, and instructions to follow up with his family doctor on Monday. The ER was empty so I went back to the call room and dropped into bed. I had been asleep for two hours when the nurses called. They had a young woman with back pain.

I staggered out of bed, pulled on my shoes, and slung my lab coat over my shoulder. I introduced myself to Mary Goff, an anxious young woman who was sitting on the edge of a cart.

"This is my husband, Jim," she said.

"Hi, Mr. Goff," I said, shaking hands with him.

Mrs. Goff then went on to describe her pain. It had started earlier that night. It didn't seem too bad at first but had slowly increased to the point to where she could hardly stand upright now.

I examined her, then ordered a blood test and a urine test. I returned a half hour later to give them the results.

"How long have you two been married?" I asked her.

"One month—today!" she answered with a little smile.

"Well," I said, "you have a bladder infection. In fact, this is a fairly common problem in newlyweds. It's called honeymoon cystitis. It's usually not serious. We'll start some antibiotics tonight. You'll need to get another urine test in a few days to be sure you're responding to treatment."

"Why is it common in newlyweds?" she asked.

"Well," I said, "when a woman isn't used to having sexual relations, sometimes a little infection can get into her bladder."

"Oh."

Mary and her husband glanced at each other and then quickly looked away. It was obvious they were uncomfortable with this discussion. It was almost as if they were embarrassed to have everyone know they had been having sex.

"Is this permanent?" she asked. "I mean, will it keep happening?"

God, the poor thing. Did she think she was going to have to give up sex or have excruciating back pain for the rest of her life?

The medical term for painful sex is dyspareunia. It seemed like an oxymoron to me. In medical school we had two weeks of sex education during our psychiatry rotation (where else would a Catholic medical school put it?). There were only two things I could remember from the entire two weeks. One was that nymphomania was not as common as my classmates and I had hoped. The other was my locker partner Joe Coyne's comment on dyspareunia. "Dyspareunia," he observed, "is better than no pareunia at all."

I turned back to Mrs. Goff. I didn't want her to think she was going to be stuck with this forever. "Usually these infections are a onetime thing," I said. "But it's important to discuss it with your gynecologist if it keeps happening."

"I don't have a . . . gynecologist." She was embarrassed to say the word.

"Well then your family doctor. Or," I said, "maybe your mother could give you some advice."

She gave me a look that said I was crazy if I thought she was going to talk to her mother about *that.*

I wrote out a couple prescriptions. "Drink lots of water," I told her. "Cranberry juice can help, too. And if you aren't getting better, come back here. Sometimes we have to use IV antibiotics if the pills don't clear up the infection."

I could see the look of horror on her face. The thought of coming back here was too much for her. I had a feeling that she was going to be drinking cranberry juice by the gallon in the next few days.

It was after six by then. I chatted with the night nurses for a while, then took a shower and shaved. Steve Tucker, who was taking over for me, came in about ten to seven.

"You survived, huh?" he said.

"Yeah. It went okay."

"Well, go home and get some sleep. It's a beautiful day."

As I walked out to the parking lot, my shaving kit under my arm, I couldn't help but feel guilty. At twenty bucks an hour, I had made almost as much money in the last twenty-four hours as I made in two weeks at Mayo. It was so much money, in so short a time. I felt like I had ripped someone off.

I grew impatient with myself. Jesus Christ, I thought, do I have to analyze everything? Who knows why moonlighters are paid more than residents. The fact is *they are.* I don't make the rules. I just live by them. I wish everyone could have free health care. I wish everyone could win the lottery. I wish the White Sox could win the World Series. Oh, and don't forget world peace and an end to hunger. Fine, okay, that's great. Now can we skip the infantile dreams and get back to reality? I moonlight so I can pay my mortgage and buy food. There is no reason to feel guilty about getting twenty dollars an hour to moonlight.

But I did.

# CHAPTER FIFTEEN

*June*

I switched off the light in the Mayo call room, adjusted the pillow, and closed my eyes. Finally! It seemed that every night I wasn't moonlighting at St. Joe's, I was on call at Mayo, and it was starting to get to me. I was nearing the end of my first year and had learned to deal with sleep deprivation, but I prayed the beeper would stay quiet for a few hours. I let out a long sigh and tried to settle in, but I couldn't. Something was wrong. I had forgotten something. What was it?

Narc rounds. I had forgotten the damned narc rounds. I slapped my pillow aside, switched on the light, and tugged on my gym shoes. "Son of a bitch!" I jerked my lab coat off the back of the chair and stomped out the door. It was twelve minutes after 3:00—A.M.

*"The order for all narcotic pain medicines must be renewed every forty-eight hours."* That was the Mayo Clinic rule and the responsibility for obeying it fell to the junior resident on call. Every night we were supposed to trudge up to the ortho floor and renew all expiring narcotic orders. If we forgot, the nurses couldn't give the patients their pain meds.

Although narc rounds were our responsibility, we assigned them a low priority. Other, more important duties often demanded our attention. We may have had to assist in surgery, or go to the ER, or admit a patient.

I usually tried to renew narcs before I went to bed, but that night I had been so busy it slipped my mind. Now it was 3:00 A.M. and I just wanted to lie down for an hour or two.

I got off the elevator and nodded to the janitor who was swishing a red scrubber back and forth across the soapy floor. "Careful, Doc," he said, nodding at the floor. I waved a hand, tiptoed through the suds, and trudged toward the nurses' station that shone like a beacon at the end of the dark, silent hall. Sure enough, when I got there I found nine charts lined up, waiting to be signed.

I had seen three consults that night, had two admissions, casted a ten-year-old kid with a broken wrist, and stitched up the leg of an old farmer who ripped his calf open on a piece of barbed wire. And now I'd been driven out of bed to perform a job a monkey could have done.

"Sign your name like a good monkey," I muttered as I began the rite of scribblage.

"Pardon me?" a nurse said. I glanced up. It was Annie Cheevers.

"Oh, nothing. I was just encouraging myself to get these charts signed."

Annie smiled pleasantly. She was used to bizarre nocturnal ramblings of junior residents—ortho dogs, we called ourselves.

Like a bored priest distributing communion I went down the line mindlessly scribbling on page after page:

> Renew narcs
>     —MJ Collins MD
> Renew narcs
>     —MJ Collins MD
> Renew narcs
>     —MJ Collins MD

I never saw the patient, never looked at the rest of the chart, never even checked the name. I just took it on faith that the nurses had pulled the correct chart and I dutifully scribbled my name.

"Good monkey," Annie said as I signed the last one.

I glared at her until I realized she was smiling sympathetically. Annie was a pleasure to look at, smart and pretty in her clean, starched nurse's uniform. Her brown hair was pulled straight back and held with a pink ribbon. She and I had by then worked together several times. With her I had started IVs, run codes, changed dressings, and fortunately only once, had to pronounce someone.

What a strange word, and an equally strange custom: to "pronounce" someone. When a patient dies it isn't good enough to say, "Yup, he's dead." A doctor, an MD, has to formally "pronounce" him dead.

Annie had paged me one night and asked me to go into a room to verify a patient's death. I entered the room, and respectfully pulled the sheet from his head. Well, I thought, he's cold, he's blue, and he's stiff. This narrows the diagnostic possibilities. To be official I felt for a carotid pulse, and then listened to the chest for a few seconds. For once the patient's chest was colder than my stethoscope.

I turned to Annie and said, "He's dead."

Annie looked at her watch. My pronouncement had to be accompanied, as in a train terminal, by the time of departure.

"Dr. Collins," Annie wrote in the chart, "pronounced the patient at 2:14 A.M."

Patti and I had both grown up in large Irish Catholic families. I was one of eight kids. She was one of seven. We were used to large weddings and larger wakes. How sad, I thought, for someone to die alone in a dark hospital room, no one holding his hand, no one shedding a tear. No one even knows he is gone until an hour later when a nurse finds him. The only notice taken of his passing is when some lowly resident, grousing and resentful, is dragged out of bed to "pronounce" him.


I leaned against the counter, resting my cheek on my fist. I had been working almost twenty hours in a row, and still had another sixteen to go. I glanced down at my rumpled lab coat, my faded scrubs with that old farmer's bloodstains on the cuffs. My mouth felt grimy, my eyes were bleary, and I needed a shave. I knew I should go to bed, but there was something refreshing about being there with Annie.

"Did you come on at eleven?" I asked, knowing full well that all night-shift nurses come on at eleven.

"Why, yes, Doctor, I did," she said, trying not to laugh.

"What's it like outside?"

"Dark," she said, nodding her head thoughtfully. "Mostly dark."

"God, it never changes around here, does it? Every night it's the same thing."

Annie smiled and began putting the charts back in the rack.

I slumped down in a chair next to her. I wanted to stay, but I couldn't think of anything to say.

"Mike," she said, a chart in her right hand, "you should get some sleep. You look terrible."

"Flattery will get you nowhere."

I sat there dumbly, too lethargic to get up.

When she finished filing the charts she said, "Okay, if you don't want to go to bed then how about seeing Mr. Flannery in twenty-three? He's got a fecal impaction. Maybe you could take care of it for him."

That did it. "All right, fine. I'll leave. But what if I never make it back to the call room? What if I collapse and die of unnatural causes at the end of some deserted hallway? It won't be so funny then, will it?" I stood up and waved my hands in the air, proclaiming the headlines:

**MAYO RESIDENT FOUND DEAD IN STORAGE ROOM. ORTHO NURSE UNDER INVESTIGATION FOR CRUELTY TO ANIMALS**

"Will you get out of here? I have work to do."

"Sure. Fine. Don't worry about me," I said as I began walking down the dark hall. "If I don't see you again, have a nice life."

"I should be so lucky."

"It'll be too late for tears when they pluck my cold, lifeless body from a floor in Central Supply."

She laughed and waved a hand at me. "Go to bed. You're nuts."

"That's what they said about Vincent van Gogh."

I trudged down the dark hall toward the elevator. My first year in orthopedic surgery was drawing to a close. I had never learned so much, never seen so much, never suffered so much as I had in this last year; and yet the road ahead seemed so long. I was still a lowly junior resident, with one more year of holding retractors, one more year of making narc rounds at three o'clock in the morning. But a spark had been ignited in me, and it enabled me to see past all the scut work and ignominy that lay ahead. In one year I would be a senior resident. In three I would be an orthopedic surgeon.

At the end of the hall, the janitor was still swishing the floor. I nodded to him, stepped gingerly across the soapy floor, and pressed the button for the elevator. I stood there, looking wrinkled, rumpled, and drained. As Frank Wales liked to say, I looked like I'd been "rode hard and put away wet." I could almost read the janitor's mind as he looked at me out of the corner of his eye. "This guy is a doctor?"

I had come so far. I had grown so much, but as I prepared to start my second year, I found myself wondering the same thing.

# YEAR TWO

# CHAPTER SIXTEEN

*July*

Although we were into our second year, we were still junior residents, still ortho dogs mired in scut work. We might open or close a case here and there, maybe remove some screws from an old ankle fracture, but none of us had done a big case.

All the fourth-year guys were gone, including Art Hestry, who had joined a practice in Vail, Colorado, and Jonathan Wilhelm—who was not asked to stay on staff at Mayo. A new crop of residents had arrived—nice guys, but as Bill Chapin said, "Were we really that green when we started?"

"I was," I said, having no illusions about how ignorant I had been just one year before.

"Yeah, I forgot. Collins, you were among the orthopedically brain dead a year ago. In fact, for a while, I think BJ Burke had you on the endangered species list. Only through the diligent efforts of Drs. Wales, Manning, and I have you started to resemble a real orthopod."

"Excuse me, but was I the resident who called the peroneal nerve the pudendal nerve?" The peroneal nerve goes to the leg. The pudendal nerve goes to the genitals. Bill had made a terrible gaffe at fracture conference last September and we had been ribbing him ever since, constantly inquiring as to the health, activity, and function of his pudendal nerve.

"For Chrissake," he muttered, "a guy makes one little mistake and his friends never let him forget it."


My first assignment of my second year was with Dr. Matt Wilk, one of Mayo's premier hand surgeons. I had been on his service for about a month when I was called to the ER to see Jason Withers, a thirty-six-year-old carpenter who had cut off all four fingers of his right hand while using a circular saw. His coworkers had enough sense to pick up the fingers, stick them in a Baggie, and put them on ice. I examined the fingers. They all looked pretty good except for the index finger, which had most of the skin and soft tissue stripped away.

I gave Jason some morphine, cultured his wounds, and started some antibiotics. Then I sent him for X-rays. I had the four amputated fingers X-rayed as well.

While we were waiting for the X-rays to come back I began talking to Jason. He was married, with two boys aged four and five.

"Doc," he said, chewing his lower lip and trying not to cry, "my hand is gone. What am I going to do? I'm a carpenter. I can't work with one hand."

I felt Jason's situation keenly. I, too, was a father with young kids. I, too, depended on my hands to make a living.

"Is there something you guys can do?" Jason asked, his eyes welling with tears. "Can you put my fingers back on?"

That was a tough call. The lacerations seemed fairly sharp. The wounds didn't appear to be grossly contaminated—but *four fingers*? That was a tall order.

The X-rays were back in ten minutes. They showed the amputation had cut across the base of the proximal phalanges of all four fingers.

I knew that not all amputated fingers could or should be reattached, but Jason seemed like a good candidate: he was young, his occupation demanded use of his hand, the injury was to his dominant hand. There was one other factor to consider, however.

"You don't smoke do you, Jason?" I asked.

"Yeah, I do."

"About how much?"

"Pack and a half, maybe two packs a day."

That complicated things. Dr. Wilk hated doing replants on smokers. The failure rate for smokers was markedly higher than the failure rate for nonsmokers. "I'm damned if I'm going to stay up all night replanting some guy's hand if he's going to turn around and wreck it all by smoking," Matt had said on more than one occasion.

"You gotta help me, Doc," Jason said. "I gotta be able to work."

This was going to be a tough sell to Dr. Wilk.

"Jason, do you think you could quit smoking?"

"Quit smoking? Yeah, I guess so, why?"

"Well, first of all because smoking is about the worst thing a man can do to his body. Second, smoking constricts blood vessels. That means *if* your fingers aren't too badly damaged, and *if* we are able to reattach them, and *if* we can get adequate blood flow to them, then all that would go down the drain if you smoked—even one cigarette. The vessels would constrict and the fingers would die."

Jason struggled to sit up in his cart. He leaned forward, reached into his shirt pocket with his left hand, took out a package of Camels, and threw them on the floor. "Doc, if you guys can put my fingers back on, I'll never smoke again, not a single cigarette. Ever."

I called Dr. Wilk and laid out the scenario for him.

"All four fingers, huh?" He thought for a moment. "Clean amputations?" he asked.

"Yeah, pretty clean."

"How long has it been since the injury occurred?" he asked.

"Two hours. And the fingers have been on ice the whole time." I was trying to convince him that we should try to replant Jason's fingers.

Dr. Wilk paused for a moment. "Sounds like a good candidate for a replant. He's not a smoker, is he?"

"Well, yeah, but he says he will quit. He says he will never take another puff."

"That's what they all say."

He remained silent until I couldn't stand it any longer.

"He's a carpenter, Dr. Wilk, and it's his dominant hand."

Still no response. Why was he being so hard-nosed?

"Sir, he's got two little kids."

"So you think we should go ahead with the replant?"

"Yes, sir. Maybe not the index finger, that looks pretty chewed up. But I think we should do the other three."

"And you believe this guy when he says he won't smoke?"

"Yes, sir. I do."

He sighed. "All right. Call the OR and let me know when they're ready."

I went back to talk to Jason. His wife had gotten there by then. I introduced myself to her. "Good news," I told them. "I talked to Dr. Wilk who is one of the world's best replant surgeons. He thinks we should try to reattach your fingers."

"Thank God," Jason said.

"Jason, don't get your hopes up too high. First of all, one of your fingers looks too bad to save. And with the other three, even if we reattach them there is no guarantee they will survive. And even if they do survive, your fingers will never be the same. They'll never work as well as they used to."

"I know, Doc. But you guys just get those fingers back on for me. I'll make 'em work."

"There is one more thing," I said. "You *have* to stop smoking." I shifted my gaze from Jason to his wife. "If he smokes, he will ruin everything. His fingers will die."

"Don't worry, Doc. If you guys can put my fingers back on I won't ever *look* at a cigarette again."

Like all replant procedures, the operation took forever. The two of us, microsurgical tools in our hands, were hunched over the operating microscope for six hours. The index finger was too badly damaged to replant, but we were able to save the other three. We anastomosed the digital vessels and nerves, repaired the tendons, and fixed the bones.

It was touch and go for the first three days. His fingers looked dark and dusky. It was hard to tell if they were going to survive. Every morning and every afternoon I would unwrap the white gauze dressings and check the fingers. They didn't look terrible, but they didn't look good.

On the morning of the fourth day, things changed. For the first time, his fingers looked a little pinker, a little healthier. On the fifth day there was no doubt: the replants were working.

Jason and his wife were thrilled. Even their untrained eyes could see the difference. With each succeeding day the fingers continued to improve. Even the therapists were amazed.

Jason went home on the tenth day after surgery. We had arranged for outpatient therapy and planned to see him back in the office in one week.

The day after he was discharged I got a frantic call from his wife. "Something happened," she said. "His fingers look awful. You have to check him right away."

I told her to bring Jason straight to the emergency room. I was waiting when they arrived. Jason's wife was right. The fingers were cold and almost black.

I was sick. "Jason," I said, "I'm so sorry. I don't know what could have happened. Something has gone wrong."

Jason didn't respond, nor did he look at me. He set his mouth in a line and stared at the ground. He looked almost guilty. A thought occurred to me.

It couldn't be, I thought. He wouldn't have been that big an idiot.

"Jason," I said, "you didn't smoke did you?"

He wouldn't answer.

I winced and shook my head in disbelief. "Oh, Jason," I said, unable to hide the disappointment and disgust I felt. It was all I could do to keep from saying, "You fucking moron."

I looked at Jason and his wife. We all knew what this meant.

"Is there anything you can do?" his wife asked.

I let out a long sigh. "I'll call Dr. Wilk. We'll have to take him back to the operating room."

She brightened slightly. "To redo the operation?"

I shook my head. "No," I said, "to see if there is anything that can be saved."


I dreaded the call to Dr. Wilk. He hadn't wanted to do the operation in the first place. I had talked him into it. I had assured him that Jason would quit smoking. All the hours of work, all the thousands of dollars expended, all our care and worry had been a waste. Jason had stuck the knife in his own back—just as Dr. Wilk suspected he would.

I couldn't believe it. I just couldn't believe it. I would have done anything for Jason. When I first met him I was so upset that he had lost his fingers that I would have given him one of my own. I had poured my heart and soul into his care. I had fretted over every little thing, trying so desperately to make the operation a success.

And the stupid idiot had ruined it all.

The more I thought of it, the angrier I became. What kind of self-destructive fool was he? Hadn't I told him fifty times not to have even one single puff? Hadn't I warned him what would happen? But he had to have his smoke, didn't he? I talked the best replant surgeon in the world into reattaching his fingers and then Jason blew it all.

Over the course of the next ten days, we brought Jason back to the OR three times, each time whittling away more and more of the necrotic tissue on his fingers until, finally, only stumps remained.

Dr. Wilk never said much. I kept waiting for the hammer to fall, waiting for him to let me know what a fool I had been, how I had wasted his and everyone else's time by insisting we reattach Jason's fingers.

I continued to see Jason twice a day, seething each time I went into his room, changing his dressings in a cold fury. I went to bat for you, my attitude said, and you betrayed me.

Finally Dr. Wilk took me aside.

Well, here it comes, I thought, the ream job of the century.

"Mike," he said, "show me your right hand."

Puzzled, I held it out to him.

"How many fingers do you have there?"

"How many . . .? Ah, four. Well, five, with my thumb."

"How many does Jason have?"

"None. Just his thumb."

"Then why don't you quit acting like *you* are the victim? Why don't you get off your high horse and start acting like a doctor, not a judge? All right, Jason did a stupid thing, but does that mean our responsibility to him is over? Do surgeons only have obligations to smart patients? Jason not only has to live without a right hand, he has to live with the knowledge that it was his own stupidity that caused it. Give the guy a break. He's suffered enough."

I gave a servile nod of the head, just as residents are supposed to do. But it took me a while to understand what Dr. Wilk had been trying to tell me. Surgeons can become too focused on surgery, too involved in the mechanics of the things they do for patients. The patient comes into *our* hospital, has *our* surgery, and follows *our* instructions. Is it any wonder that we fall into the trap of thinking that their injury is actually *our* injury, of wanting the patient not to get in the way of the management of our problem?

It's not about the problem, and it's not about the surgeon, Dr. Wilk was telling me. It's about a human being who needs our help, not our judgment.

I wasn't sure what to say to Jason. When I changed his dressing the following morning I told him I was sorry things had turned out the way they did.

"And I'm sorry for not being more understanding," I said to him. "I know you wouldn't have smoked if you knew what was going to happen."

Jason didn't reply for a while, then in a low voice he said, "I know it doesn't matter now. I know I'm a fucking cripple for life, but . . ." He set his jaw and gave me a fierce, determined look. "I'm going to quit smoking. I'll never have another goddamn cigarette for the rest of my life."

Too little, too late? I didn't think so. It was a start. There would be time to deal with the self-pity and self-loathing later. We would start occupational therapy. We would arrange for vocational rehab. It was too late to get his hand back, but we could still help him get a life.

"That's a good first step, Jason," I said.

# CHAPTER SEVENTEEN

*August*

Sometimes the life of a junior resident got to be too much. At 6:45 one Tuesday morning, Jack Manning looked up from the sports section of the *Post-Bulletin*. "You know," he said, "this sucks." He closed the paper and slid it away from him. "This whole thing sucks."

"You talking about the French toast?" Bill asked.

"No, asshole. I mean this." He looked around the room, waving his hands at everything and nothing. "All this bullshit we have to go through." He set his dirty glasses on the table and rubbed his bloodshot eyes. "I was up the whole damn night—"

A chorus of sarcastic "Ooohhhs" arose from the rest of the table. "Poor baby," Bill said. Jack was talking to the wrong crowd if he wanted sympathy.

Jack ignored the interruption. "I didn't even get to see my bed. I was up all night doing stupid shit any janitor could have done." He reached over and took the cup of coffee from Bill's tray.

"And it wouldn't be so bad if I was doing something worthwhile, but all I did was narc rounds and start about ten IVs, then go sew up some drunken biker dude's leg. The dumb shit drove through the front window of the flower shop across the street. Never even slowed down. When the cops got there his bike was still running and he was passed out in a pile of carnations with his leg bleeding like stink. The whole floor was covered with blood. His hemoglobin was eight when we got him in the ER.

"And the whole time I'm sewing up his leg, he's telling me what a pussy I am and how he's gonna kick my ass as soon as we let him out of restraints, which, if I have my way, will be in about six years." He sighed and took a tentative sip of the coffee he was holding in both hands.

"Then I got stuck babysitting one of Hale's patients who kept saying that her pain was so bad it was like a million atom bombs exploding in her vagina."

Bill coughed up a mouthful of orange juice. "So, Dr. Freud, did you explore the implications of this metaphor with her?"

"It wasn't a metaphor. It was a simile, and no I didn't. She said she was going insane and she wanted me to call Hale at home and get him to come in."

"Yeah, he'da loved that," Bill said, reaching for the crumpled sports section.

"Who's got atom bombs in her vagina?" Frank asked, putting his tray down and squeezing in with us.

"Don't ask," Bill said. "Manning is rambling on about his night on call."

Jack ignored the interruption. "Then," he said, "some lady up on Seven had chest pain . . ." He hung his head and shook it wearily. "And every ten minutes someone else would call me to go start another IV. Hell, I musta started ten of 'em."

"Yeah, yeah. You already told us that," Bill said, without looking up from the paper.

"And you know what else I'm sick of?" Jack asked. "I'm sick of having all the patients think that I am nothing but a fucking spear carrier for the almighty attending. I do all the work. I admit 'em. I do the H&P. I start their IV when no one else can. I do every lousy job in the book. And every single person in this hospital thinks I'm shit—attendings, nurses, patients, all of them.

"Well, the next time one of the nurses calls me I'm going to admit I'm shit. I'll just walk in the patient's room and introduce myself. 'Howdy, ma'am, I'm here to start your IV. I have to do it because Dr. Farthingham, your *real* doctor, is out playing golf. I do all the shit jobs.'

"And she'll say, 'What is your name, tall stranger?'

"And I'll look her right in the eye and say, 'Shit. Joe Shit. At your service, ma'am.'

"But I won't get discouraged. I'll work and I'll slave. I'll do all those jobs no one else will do. And someday, somehow, I'll finish my residency, and I'll open a posh practice in Manhattan with scribbly paintings and Navajo rugs on the wall. And I'll hire some supermodel as a receptionist. Of course I'll have to change my name. Joe Shit won't cut it in Manhattan. I'll get a gold-plated sign outside my paneled door: Joseph Faeces, MD."

Bill yawned. "Yeah, that's great, Jack, or Joe, or whatever your name is. I'll be sure to send lots of patients to you."

Conversation continued at the tables around us, but we were silent until Jack started up again.

"I'm telling you, this sucks."

No one cared. What was the point of talking about it? Nothing was going to change. We just had to deal with it. Complaining didn't help.

Jack slammed Bill's now-empty coffee cup on the table. "Listen," he said, "we don't have to put up with this shit. We can change our residency. After all, who knows more about residencies than residents? We can go to the Clinic and demand they look into this."

The rest of us shifted in our seats and looked at each other. What was Jack's problem? There's good and bad in everything, and things here weren't that bad. It sure wasn't worth starting some big revolt. And Jack seemed like that last guy you would pick to be a rabble-rousing agitator. He just had a bad night on call, that's all.

"I want to know that you guys support me," he said. "I want to go to BJ and give him a list of demands. I want to tell him how this residency should be run."

"What are you going to do for a living after BJ fires your ass?" Bill said.

The rest of us remained puzzled. We'd never seen Jack so worked up. Was he trying to get himself booted out of the program?

Jack stood up and slapped the paper out of Bill's hands. "Listen to me!" he said wildly. "We're going to change things. We're going to change them starting right here, right now. No more fucking narc rounds. No more starting IVs in the middle of the night."

His voice was rising. Residents at surrounding tables were starting to listen, wondering what was going on.

"I've had it!" he roared. "This is all going to change. And the first thing that's going to change is call. *I'm not taking any more call!*" He was shouting now and the entire cafeteria was listening. Medical students in line gaped in amazement. Nurses with plates of food stopped and stared.

"Starting today," Jack said, "ortho call will be taken only by attendings. IVs will be started only by Clinic administrators. Narc rounds will be performed by emeritus staff and must be done between three and four in the morning."

People started laughing. We ortho residents breathed a sigh of relief. Jack was on a roll. He stood up on his chair and started appealing to the faces around him. "Your Attention Please. This is the revolt of the ortho dogs! We wish to inform you that the Mayo Clinic Orthopedic Junior Residency will now take place in the south of France. The assigned hours will be Tuesday through Thursday from ten A.M. until four P.M. Noontime clinical conferences will take place over bottles of chilled champagne and imported oysters."

We were all clapping and laughing. Frank let out a cowboy, "Eeeh-hah!"

Jack was shouting now to be heard over the laughter. "All nurses," he said, "will be named Babette or Cherie and will be required to have extremely large breasts which they will cover with only the flimsiest of material. They will also be highly skilled in the arts of massage and yoga."

"Yeah! And what about getting rid of our beepers?" someone shouted.

"Don't be an idiot," Jack sneered at him. "We will need the beepers so the chef can let us know when the Roast Duckling Montmorency with flaming cherry sauce is ready."

The crowd roared its approval with each new declaration. From behind the polished serving counters, women in hairnets, serving spoons in their hands, looked on in amusement. Janitors in faded blue overalls leaned on their mops, and smiled as the tirade continued.

"At the completion of their training program all residents will undergo extensive testing. Those with insufficiently high liver enzymes or inappropriately low levels of prostatic hypertrophy will be forced to remain for further training."

He raised his hands and silenced the crowd. "Gentlemen," he said, looking down at the table of ortho residents at his feet, "this offer is good for a limited time only. Please have your applications on my desk in the morning." Then he raised his eyes and looked at the internists around us. "Fleas need not apply."

A chorus of boos and a hail of napkins and pieces of toast greeted him from the surrounding tables. He covered his head and quickly sat down. Within a few seconds everyone had turned away. The line started moving again. The janitors resumed their mopping. Two medical students who had been with us for the last week came over and timidly asked if they could sit with us. Jack reached over and removed a cup of coffee from one of their trays. He leaned back and sighed. "It's a dog's life, boys," he said. "It's a dog's life."

# CHAPTER EIGHTEEN

*September*

I moonlighted about two weekends a month at St. Joe's. On the other weekends I was usually on call at Mayo. This meant I would sometimes work fourteen to twenty-one days in a row before I had a day off. Whenever I had a little free time I tried to spend it with Patti and the kids.

I made rounds early one Saturday morning, then we drove up to St. Paul to see my brother Pete who was a student at St. Thomas College. We had a picnic, watched a Disney movie, and finished the day with dinner at a nice Italian restaurant that had singing waiters. Finally, around 9:00 P.M. we piled the kids into the backseat and headed home.

An oldies station was playing softly as we headed south on Highway 52 to Rochester. It was dark in the car. The kids were asleep in their car seats, their heads lolling forward, teddy bears clutched in their hands and blankets tucked around them.

We drove for a while and then Patti asked, "What Mass should we go to tomorrow?"

Oh, God, I thought, I must have forgotten to tell her. "Patti," I said as gently as I could, "I'm moonlighting tomorrow."

"Oh, Mike," she said. Her words were a groan of weariness and disappointment, frustration and irritation, betrayal and oppression. "I was hoping for once we could . . ."

She raised her hands weakly and let them fall in her lap. I could see the light from the oncoming headlights reflecting off her tears. I couldn't bear the note of hopelessness in her voice.

I was starting to hate myself and the things I did to the woman I loved. I reached for her hand. She started to pull away, then relented. The motion made the front seat rock back and forth.

"It's not my fault," I said. It sure as hell was my fault, and I knew it. "It's just that, well, I don't know what we would do if I didn't moonlight."

"Oh, I know," she said in a choked little voice.

She knew. She didn't like it any more than I did, but she knew I had no more control over my life than she had over hers. We did what we had to do. She unbuckled her seat belt, slid over, took my arm in hers, and laid her head against my shoulder.

An hour later when I pulled into our driveway in Rochester they were all asleep.


By 6:30 the next morning I had finished rounds and was halfway to Mankato. Mine was the only car on the road, a green tank rumbling westward through the rolling farms and woods of southeastern Minnesota; my only company, the ragged strands of geese winging low over the fields, heading south. I had the window down, loving the smell of the farms and the coolness of the early morning. I crested a long hill and saw tall fields of corn, punctuated by thick stands of oak and elm, stretching as far as I could see. The sun was just coming up in my rearview mirror, and patches of gray mist were lingering over the low, wet fields where the pheasant rose.

Periodically the speed limit would drop to thirty as I passed through small towns—Waseca, Janesville, Smith's Mill. I would take my foot off the accelerator and coast down the three-block-long stretch of Main Street. In each town the only thing open was the small diner with three or four old Ford pickups parked in front. Inside, men in faded, blue overalls and green John Deere caps sat hunched at the counter over coffee and eggs.

I envied them. I envied their easy familiarity, their taken-for-granted intimacy. I was nothing but a hired gun caring for a succession of strangers whose lives would briefly touch mine and then swing away forever. I wasn't Mike Collins to them. I was "the guy in the ER who casted my ankle," or "that ER doc, the one from Mayo, who stitched up my leg." If I ran into one of them on the street it is doubtful they would even recognize me.

But I longed to connect with the people I treated. I wanted to be more than just the dispensing machine that gave them their pills when they put in their quarter. I wanted to walk into one of those diners and be recognized and welcomed.

The bell over the door would tinkle as I came in. The guys at the counter would turn around and greet me as I hung my coat on the hook in the corner.

"Hey, Doc."

"Mornin', Doc."

Steve, behind the counter, would smile and pour me some coffee as I swung my leg over the stool. Arnie, sitting next to me, would push back his hat and ask if I could believe the North Stars hadn't pulled their goalie last night with a minute left and the face-off in the Maple Leafs zone.

We'd all shake our heads in disbelief.

"Cold this morning," I would say as I wrapped my hands around my mug of coffee.

Steve, returning to the grill where he was tossing a pile of hash browns, would nod and say, "Yup. I hear they had frost up on the Range last night."


When I reached the end of town I jabbed at the accelerator. What was the point of this daydreaming? I wasn't getting up at 4:30 in the morning and driving halfway across the state just so I could be someone's pal. I wasn't Albert Schweitzer or Francis of Assisi. I was just a broke resident who needed money. I was a businessman engaged in a commercial transaction. And the people I treated, they weren't looking for a new friend. They just wanted someone to make their earache go away or to sew up the cut on their forehead. I should just do my work, take my paycheck, and go home. I was a businessman. Period.

Maybe. But I kept thinking there was another name for what I was doing, another name for someone who sold himself.


At nine o'clock that morning a thirty-eight-year-old man with a scraggly mustache and a three-day growth of beard came in. He was leaning on a friend. "Walt's been sick," the friend said. "He's been throwing up and I think he's getting dehydrated."

The nurses and I helped him to a cart. "Mr. . . ." I looked at the chart. "Mr. Delfmeier? I'm Dr. Collins."

"You can call me Walt," the man said. "Mr. Delfmeier is my dad."

While the nurses were getting his vitals I examined him. He was an obese man, with diffuse, but mild tenderness in the belly. He was breathing rapidly, almost gasping for breath. At first I thought he was winded from climbing up on the cart, but when the heavy breathing continued I became suspicious.

"Do you have diabetes, Walt?" I asked.

"Nope."

I ordered some blood gases and labs. Walt, meanwhile, kept falling asleep. I continued to wake him periodically to ask questions. He was friendly and cooperative.

Thirty minutes later I got the results of the blood tests. The normal blood glucose level for a healthy person is around one hundred. Walt's glucose was "greater than 900," which was as high as the machine in the lab could measure. The tech later diluted the specimen and called back to say that his glucose level was 1443, which was the highest blood glucose level I had ever seen—or heard of.

His blood gases came back several minutes later. They showed that Walt was in diabetic ketoacidosis. I pushed some fluid, gave him some insulin, and called the internist on call. Walt then started vomiting a dark-colored emesis that tested positive for blood.

I was making the arrangements for Walt to be admitted to the ICU when

Dr. Whitson, the internist, called back. He said Walt didn't need to go to the ICU. "Just send him to a regular bed on the medical floor," Whitson said.

I told him I was uncomfortable with that decision. Walt was conscious and his vitals were stable, but the guy seemed like a powder keg to me.

Dr. Whitson resented being second-guessed. "How many diabetics have you taken care of?" he asked.

"I'm an orthopod," I said, "but I still think—"

"Send him to the floor." He hung up.

That was the last I heard of Walt until 2:30 that morning when the code call came over the loudspeaker: "430! 430! 430!" It was the responsibility of the ER doctor to respond to all in-house emergencies so I sprinted up the stairs to room 430 where two nurses were already doing CPR on a man. It took me a few seconds to realize it was Walt.

I told them to hold CPR for a moment while I checked his pulse. The EKG leads were on so I checked his rhythm, as well. At that point I noticed that some kind of liquid was running from the side of his mouth. I grabbed his shoulder and tilted him to the side. A frightening amount of black fluid gushed out. Great puddles of it ran across the bed and down to the floor, spattering my pants and shoes.

Once I had his airway reasonably clear I inserted an ET tube into his trachea, and then an NG tube into his stomach. The black fluid had to be blood so I ordered up four units of blood from the lab.

Dr. Whitson arrived a few minutes later and took command of the code. We did not speak to each other. Since Whitson was there, I was free to go, but I stayed on, hoping for a miracle.

There were eight of us crammed into that little room, but it remained unusually quiet. The fact that this was a thirty-eight-year-old man weighed heavily on us. We all realized the enormity of the tragedy. The room was a mess. There was black blood all over the floor, red blood all over the bed where Whitson had tried to get in a central line. Tubes and sponges were scattered everywhere.

Twenty minutes later a nurse came up and said the emergency room needed me. I told Whitson I had to leave. He glanced over at me and nodded. His look told me what I already knew: Walt wasn't going to make it.

As I trudged back to the ER I passed a patient standing in the door of his room. He obviously had been listening to everything that had been going on. He looked at me and said hi.

Of all the things that happened that night, it was that patient's look and greeting that most sticks in my mind. The look, just the look, said so much more than he or I could ever have articulated. There was admiration in it, a bit of gratitude, and a lot of sympathy. It was as though he knew my weariness, my bewilderment, my dejection, and having sensed those things, he was telling me it was okay. I had done my best, and it was okay.

I wonder if there really was such a message sent to me by that patient in the door, or if I saw in his look what I wanted to see. Did I merely imagine the solace and comfort I so sorely needed? It is hard to tell. When a tragedy like that is unfolding you desperately want to believe you can make a difference. You convince yourself you can alter the course of events around you.

And then it is all over. A thirty-eight-year-old man who was living and breathing and talking to you sixteen hours ago is now cooling in a puddle of his own blood; and you, who so desperately tried to convince yourself that you could make a difference, must now ask yourself why you didn't. Is it because you were up against the inevitable all along and no doctor anywhere could have made a difference? Or is it because you didn't do *this,* or you should have done *that*, or you didn't consider *this*, or you neglected to see *that*?

You are left to conclude that you are either a blind fool who couldn't recognize the inevitable when he saw it, or you are an incompetent idiot who had a chance to save a life and blew it.

It's not much of a choice, but there it is. There is your late-night menu for you. Thank God for the mind-numbing weariness that leaves you unable to engage in such introspection. You do your work and when you're done, you lay your head on a pillow. But, while you wait for sleep to come, the ghosts of all your whirling memories vie for possession of your fading consciousness. They are patient, those ghosts, and if they don't have their say tonight, they have a way of returning nights or years later.

There is no resolution to these conflicts. The questions are fashioned in a manner that defies answering. It is torment these questions are meant to evoke, not answers. What happened? Why did it happen? Why were you involved in it? Why did you fail? How can you stand it? How can any good man, any feeling man, stand it? Don't you care? Don't you have any feelings?

Perhaps that is why I needed to arm myself with memories like the look of that man in the door, the look in which I thought I saw sympathy and admiration.

Back in the ER there were six patients, all of them upset at having to wait so long, all of them certain I had been sleeping or watching *Saturday Night Live* reruns. Connie Fritz, the charge nurse, tried to hand me a chart, but I brushed past her and went back to the call room. I took off my black-spattered lab coat and dropped it in one of the laundry baskets. Then I went into the bathroom to wash the blood off my hands.

It seemed to take a long time.

# CHAPTER NINETEEN

*October*

On a quiet Saturday afternoon I was in the call room at St. Joe's studying. My eyes were closed. My breathing was slow and regular. Rockwood and Green's textbook on fractures was lying on my chest. I was trying to transdermally absorb the chapter on supracondylar fractures. My studying was interrupted by the ringing of the phone.

"Hello," I mumbled.

It was Marcie from the ER. "Dr. Collins," she said, "we've got a patient here who refuses to speak to anyone but the doctor."

I'd been down that road before. It was usually some guy with gonorrhea. They never wanted to talk to the nurses. As I stood up the book fell to the floor. I sighed and ran a hand through my hair. When I got to the ER, Marcie shrugged her shoulders and handed me a chart: Mark Spahn, twenty-three years old.

I pulled back the curtain and entered his cubicle. "Hi, Mr. Spahn. I'm Dr. Collins."

He looked at me but said nothing.

"Mr. Spahn, is there something I can help you with?"

He shifted on the cart and glanced around him uncomfortably. He mumbled something unintelligible.

"Mr. Spahn, would you like to go into one of the private rooms?"

He shot me a look of gratitude. "Yeah, Doc, I would."

We went into Room Four, the gyne room, where we did pelvic exams. I closed the door.

"Now," I said, "what can I do for you?"

"It's like this, Doc," he said, refusing to look at me. "I, uh . . . well, I . . ."

"You what?"

He put his hand over his mouth, as if trying to keep the words from coming out. He looked at the floor, and in a barely audible voice, the words tumbled out. "Igotadildoupmyass."

"You got a *what*?" It took me a second or two to realize what he had said. "Oh," I replied calmly, as though this were a common problem. (*"How was your day, dear?" "Oh, the usual. Just a few guys with dildos up their asses."*)

"How did this happen, Mr. Spahn?"

"Well"—he sighed and rubbed the back of his neck—"I was just sticking it up there, and it went in too far. I couldn't get it out. I even gave myself an enema and it still wouldn't come out."

(*Don't you hate it when that happens?*)

I did a quick physical exam to make sure he didn't have any peritoneal signs and then sent him to X-ray. Fifteen minutes later he was back and, sure enough, the X-ray showed a big old dildo sitting right there in his rectum. A crowd of techs, nurses, and secretaries were gathered around the view box staring at the X-ray. I gave them a dirty look and they pretended to do other things. I went back to Mr. Spahn.

"Yep," I said, "it's there all right." I had him lie down while I did a rectal exam. I could just barely feel the tip of it. This, I thought, is nothing I want to mess with.

I phoned the general surgeon on call. He did not seem particularly empathetic. He groaned and told me to give the patient an enema. I wasn't too keen on that idea since I thought it would drive the dildo deeper inside, but I told the nurses to give him an enema.

It drove the dildo deeper inside.

I called the surgeon back. He said, "Goddamn it," and told me he would be there in five minutes. A half hour later he came in and fished around in the kid's rectum with a uterine tenaculum for ten or fifteen minutes. Finally he came out of the room red-faced, mumbling about "this stupid bullshit." He told me he couldn't get the damned thing out and I should call Rochester and ship him to Mayo.

I didn't like that idea, either. If we shipped the kid to Mayo, I would have to call there and identify myself as the transferring physician. Over the past year my reputation in the department had been growing, and the last thing I needed was for BJ Burke to read the transfer sheet and think Mike Collins was moonlighting in Mankato as a dildo extractor.

I called St. Mary's and asked for the general surgery resident on call. Thank God it was Jerry Washburn, my old partner from the ERSS.

"Hey, Jer," I said, "it's Mike Collins. I'm in Mankato and I have a patient to transfer to you."

"Oh, no," he groaned, "not another one."

I had more than my share of big-time trauma when I was moonlighting, and it seemed every time I called them I was sending them another train wreck.

"Relax," I said. "For once I've got a simple one for you."

"What's that mean, the heart's still beating for a change?"

"No. I mean it. It's just a guy with a foreign body."

"In his trachea?"

"Well, not exactly." I cleared my throat. "Actually it is lodged in another orifice."

There was a long pause at the other end. "Jesus Christ, Collins, where do you get these cases?"

"Listen," I told him. "This is an emergency. You've gotta move on this guy. He's gotta get to the big medical center where they have specialists in rectal foreign bodies. Be a good boy and page the Emergency Dildo Extracting Service. Tell them to get an OR ready."

Jerry said he would get me for this. He said the state of Minnesota wasn't big enough to hide me.

I told him we were wasting valuable time. "Every second counts," I said. "What if his batteries run down before we get him to you?"

"Collins," he said, "somewhere, somehow, I am going to find the skuzziest ortho case in the history of medicine. I'm going to wait until you are chief resident (assuming they are crazy enough to make you one) and I am going to send it to you. At three o'clock in the morning. On Christmas. When your wife is nine months pregnant. For the tenth time."

"Have a nice day, Doctor," I told him.

My first exposure to sexually aberrant practices had been in medical school. I was leafing through a textbook on forensic pathology when I came across a chapter on deviant sexual behavior. Like any red-blooded, twenty-four-year-old male I was immediately interested. We were on to something here. Intracellular accumulation of complex lipids would have to wait. I grabbed a beer and a bag of pretzels and sat down for some serious studying. I opened the chapter and immediately came across a category of behavior intriguingly labeled: "Acts Abhorrent to Nature."

Hmm. Sounds interesting.

The first section in the chapter was labeled *Necrophilia*. Necrophilia? The ensuing discussion made no attempt to define the term, assuming any intelligent reader would know what it meant. *This* reader did not know, so I turned to my ever-present *Stedman's Medical Dictionary* for help. "Necrophilia: the practice of engaging in sexual intercourse with a dead body."

I stared at the page in disbelief, my eyes bulging, my mouth gaping. "With a dead body? *A dead body?*" Not only had I never heard of it, I couldn't imagine it. Maybe *one* person, *one* time, in the entire history of the world might have been sick enough to do such a thing, but I couldn't believe there actually was a name for it. It was like having a name for albino midgets who lick purple doorknobs. I mean, come on, how many can there be?

I was still shaking my head in amazement that night after our softball game. We were standing at the bar in O'Dea's pub on West Division Street, ten or fifteen young, mostly Irish Catholic guys from the West Side of Chicago. None of us very, if at all, experienced sexually.

"Honest to God, you guys," I said. "It means someone who goes around screwing dead bodies."

There was a chorus of disbelief. "Aw, bullshit," they all replied. "Don't you doctors have anything better to do than sit around and make up stories about perverts?"

"No, I swear. It's right there in the dictionary: 'sexual intercourse with a corpse.'"

"Is this what our young people are being taught in school?" said another. "No wonder our country is going to the dogs. Oh, by the way," he went on innocently, "if you screw a dead dog is that bestiality or necrophilia?"

"It's true love," said another.

It was too fantastic, too unimaginable—and therefore, perfectly ripe for humor. Our shortstop pushed back his chair and began limping across the floor, pretending to drag a corpse behind him. "You guys make me sick," he said. "Why can't you leave us alone?

"Just say 'no,' if you want me to stop, sweetie," he said tenderly to his imaginary corpse.

By that point I realized I never should have mentioned the subject.

But my enlightenment in matters of perversion was not at an end. The next section in my forensic path book was entitled pedophilia. Pedophilia? I mused. What the hell is that? I thought back to my high school Latin. *Pes, pedis*—feet.

Feet? I thought in astonishment. What do they do with feet? I thought I must be the biggest babe in the woods in the history of North America.

After reading about sex with corpses I was ready to believe anything. I tried to picture some unshaven man in a dirty trench coat performing all kinds of fantastic acts with his feet.

It was getting to be too much for me. Maybe this medical school thing wasn't such a good idea after all. Corpses, feet. What the hell was next, sex with fish? Sex with dead fish? Sex with dead fishes' feet?

In dismay I turned again to *Stedman's Dictionary.* I don't know if I was relieved or appalled when I learned that pedophilia was not sex with feet, but sex with children. At least I'd heard of the latter.

I finally got Mr. Spahn shipped off to Rochester. He objected to being sent in an ambulance, but I wasn't taking the chance of his colon perforating if he stopped at home and tried to get it out with a coat hanger.

I saw Jerry Washburn at breakfast a few days later. "So, Jer, whatever happened to that guy with the dildo? Did you get it out okay?"

"The dedicated general surgeons at the Mayo Clinic performed yet another medical miracle. We gently and lovingly removed the young man's device. It was then sterilized, disinfected, and returned to its rightful owner none the worse for wear."

"Good. Now I know who to call if I get another one."

He put down his forkful of scrambled eggs and leaned across the table. "Don't do me any favors, okay?"

# CHAPTER TWENTY

*November*

I was the junior resident on call at St. Mary's when they brought Ben in. There wasn't much anyone could have done for him. He was probably dead before they loaded him in the back of the pickup. At least that's what I kept telling myself.

And I kept thinking foolish things. I kept feeling guilty that while his arm was getting torn off I was lying on a couch in the residents' lounge reading Louis L'Amour. Why? What possible reason did I have to feel guilty?

I don't know, maybe it wasn't guilt. Maybe it was frustration that we couldn't help him, that our best wasn't good enough. Or maybe it was resentment that life isn't all smiles, and surgeons aren't always successful, and sometimes the bad guys win.

He was only sixteen. I learned later that he and his three brothers had been bringing in the corn on their father's farm near Kasson when the sleeve of Ben's blue jean jacket got caught in the power take-off. He must have turned and brushed against it. One second he was fine, the next he was yanked sideways, flipped over the power take-off, and slammed head-first to the ground. His body wedged under the wheels of the tractor, and as the power take-off kept spinning, his left arm was tensioned terribly, then torn from its socket with a sucking, popping sound. Blood began spurting from the gaping wound at his shoulder.

The other boys stared, first at their brother's body and then at his arm, caught in the power take-off, spinning round and round, spraying blood everywhere, making a rapid *phlap-phlap-phlap-phlap* noise as it hit the ground with each revolution.

Evan, the youngest, was the first to reach Ben. He stopped short of the body, as though afraid to approach it. "Ben?" he said tentatively. His two older brothers pushed Evan aside and knelt down next to Ben.

Norman turned him over. "Oh, Jesus, Ben," he said, leaning forward to touch his cheek. Ben's eyes were closed. The top of his head was swollen. He wasn't moving.

Donald scrambled to his feet, leaned over, and shut down the tractor. Ben's arm made one last *phlap* sound as it hit the ground. Then it dangled obscenely from the greasy metal coupling. Blood was pumping steadily from the gaping hole in Ben's shoulder. Norman tried to smother it with his hand, but the blood leaked through his fingers.

"Shit," Donald said, watching the blood pour from Ben's arm socket. "He's gonna bleed to death if we don't get him to a hospital."

He and Norman lifted Ben and carried him to the pickup. They set him down in the dirt while they dropped the tailgate, clambered onto the bed, and heaved the four bales of hay over the side. In the distance the boys could see their father's tractor moving silently up and back through the north field a half mile away.

"Evan!" Donald shouted. "Go tell Dad what happened. Tell him we're going to take Ben to St. Mary's."

Evan was still standing next to the spot where Ben had been thrown. He was staring at the dark spot in the dirt at his feet. He looked first at one brother, then the other. He seemed not to have heard.

"Evan, goddamn it, go tell Dad!"

Evan jerked suddenly and began running toward the north field. "Dad! Dad!" He was screaming and waving his arms as he ran. Norman and Donald lifted the body of their brother into the back of the pickup.

"You stay with Ben." Donald said. "I'll drive." He vaulted over the side and sprinted back to the power take-off. He pulled tentatively on the mangled arm entwined around the dirty shaft. It wouldn't come free. He pulled again, more forcefully this time, but it still wouldn't come loose. Finally, he took his jackknife and cut away the sleeve. He carried the arm back to the pickup and laid it on the seat next to him. Norman meanwhile had hooked his right arm over the side of the truck. With his left arm he lifted Ben's head and cradled it in his lap.

"Oh, Jesus, Ben," he kept repeating.

Donald rammed the truck into gear and it lurched forward, spraying gravel and manure from the rear wheels. Norman was flung first backward, then forward as the truck shot out of the farmyard.

The ER had no clue they were coming. Donald pulled right up to the ambulance entrance. He ran in, holding Ben's bloody arm in his left hand, and started yelling that he needed help, that his brother was "hurt bad."

John Stevenson, who was on ortho trauma call, Joe Stradlack from the ERSS, and Jeannie Popp, the head ER nurse, saw him waving the bloody arm. They ran out to the truck where Norman, tears running silently down his cheeks, was still sitting in the back of the pickup, stroking Ben's hair. They loaded Ben onto a gurney and wheeled him into Trauma One.

I was up in the call room when my beeper went off. "Dr. Collins, please call the ER, 5591, 5591, 5591. Please call the ER, STAT, 5591."

They don't say *stat* in the ER unless they mean it, so I immediately picked up the phone. "Code in Trauma One," I was told. "Kid with a power take-off injury."

I threw my book aside and sprinted down the stairs. I got there just as Joe finished putting in the subclavian line. I glanced at the monitor over the bed and saw the patient had no rhythm. Then I saw he had no arm.

The nurses were squeezing O-negative blood into him as fast as they could. John Stevenson was fishing around in the bloody stump of the axilla with a hemostat looking for something to clamp, but by then the kid didn't have much blood left anyway.

We went to work. We pumped him full of blood, shot him full of drugs, flailed away with CPR, clamped and cauterized various unrecognizable strands of vessels in the stump. All the while his skin kept growing colder, and doughier, and bluer. John and I kept looking at Joe out of the corner of our eyes, wondering, waiting, thanking God it was his call, not ours. Finally, when we had done everything we could think of, twice, Joe slowly straightened up and tossed a bloody wad of 4×4s on the kid's chest.

"That's it," he said.

The code nurse asked, "Are you calling the code, Doctor?"

I wanted to shout, "What the hell do you *think* he's doing?" but Joe just said quietly, "Yes, I'm calling the code."

As usual, I had no time to think about what had just happened. For the next eight hours there were lacerations to sew up, consults to see, fractures to set. At 4:00 A.M. I wrapped the last bit of plaster around the leg of the seventeen-year-old girl in the car crash, wrote out her prescription, and dutifully recited the fracture care instructions to her parents.

I took the elevator to the sixth floor and walked down the silent corridor to the call room. I shouldered the door open. It banged against the opposite wall and slowly swung shut behind me. The wooden chair scraped across the marble floor as I pulled it from under the desk. I dropped into the chair and closed my eyes. It was quiet up here, away from the patients and machines. It was nice to sit with my mind turned off for a while. I slumped back in the chair, thankful for the silence. Somewhere down the hall, a door opened and closed. I heard the steady click of footsteps approaching and then gradually fading in the distance.

My shaving kit was sitting on the desk where I had left it twenty-one hours before. The room was immaculate. The cleaning ladies had come around in the morning after everyone left for surgery or rounds. At that time of day, the rooms were always a mess. Newspapers, call schedules, notes, and lists littered the floor. Wet towels lay in a heap in the corner of the bathroom, or hung limply from the back of a chair. The rooms often were dirtier than they had to be, almost as though the residents, tired of feeling abused, tired of cleaning up other people's messes, had decided to abuse someone else, to create a mess for someone else to clean up.

I had never seen the cleaning ladies. I had never been in the call room when they were around. There was just too much to do. While we stitched up wounds, assisted at surgery, or set fractures, the cleaning ladies swept floors, changed sheets, and washed the sink and shower. They scooped up the disordered pile of books and arranged them tidily with Charnley's *Closed Treatment of Common Fractures,* two old anatomy books, and the aged copy of Campbell's *Operative Orthopedics* neatly stacked on their sides propping up a long row of well-worn Louis L'Amour paperbacks.

The sheets and gray woolen blanket were tucked tight and crisp under the mattress. The doors, the walls, the desk, the square metal ends of the bed, all rose and intersected at their perfect right angles. Everything was so symmetric, so defined. Sometimes, coming back to this room late at night, the cleanliness, the order, and the symmetry would comfort me. But not tonight. Tonight the incongruity of it all overwhelmed me.

Everything inside me seemed to have been beaten away. I wasn't tired. I wasn't depressed. I wasn't sad, or outraged, or horrified. I was just empty. I kept seeing the gaping hole where Ben's shoulder should have been. I kept feeling guilty that Ben's death was another step on my learning curve, another item on my résumé. I needed things like that to become a surgeon. They brought me a step closer to my goal.

The whole thing made me sick. I wondered if any goal could be worth all this. It wasn't that I minded the work. In some ways the mind-numbing drudgery was my salvation. It was a crutch, a shield. I got tied up in it and it insulated me, protected me. It used me, but I used it, too; and I had drifted into a comfortable marriage with it. I immersed myself in work in order to distort and disguise what I did.

That was not a human being my scalpel was slicing through. It was a knee. No, not a knee but a meniscus. No, not a meniscus but a target, a single unit of focus upon which my attention could be riveted. It was like one of those sequences of pictures from outer space where first we saw the North American continent wedged between two vast oceans, then we zoomed down to New England, then to Vermont, then finally to the little town of Mapleton where, in the backyard of that Victorian house on Elmwood Avenue there was a dark red picnic table upon which a baked potato lay steaming. The larger context was irrelevant. The locus of the potato was inconsequential. At that precise moment there was nothing outside the framework of the lens.

A young boy slipped and got his arm caught in a power take-off. He came to the ER with a gaping hole where his arm used to be. How much easier it was to focus on some specific thing: his hypovolemia, his lytes, where we would take the vein graft, what kind of ex-fix to use. We are not meant to see sixteen-year-old kids die. We are not meant to see arms ripped out of sockets.

My bloody hand, removing the last shred of Ben's brachial plexus, was neither bloody nor mine. The plexus was neither severed nor brachial. It was merely a white target in a red-black hole. I could avoid the implications of my actions by ignoring the context in which they took place. They were isolated acts, devoid of meaning or greater significance. But I couldn't deceive myself forever. The hand that emerged from that gaping wound was not the hand that had entered it, and the eyes that finally turned away from that mangled corpse were not the eyes that first registered the gory scene.

I picked up my shaving kit and walked into the bathroom where I brushed my teeth and splashed some water on my face. As I dried myself I held the towel against my eyes for a few seconds, then draped it over the sink. I had no interest in seeing the face in the mirror.

Why couldn't I just take things as they came? Why was I continually looking for reasons and meaning? Reasons and meaning are not pragmatic. They are not the stuff of residencies. BJ Burke was not interested in what I thought or understood. He was interested in what I did.

"If you want to learn to be sensitive and introspective," he would say, "do it on your own time."

I imagined myself being called into his office. As I enter the room he is seated at his desk, reading the report in front of him. He makes certain I know I am being ignored.

At length he looks at me over the top of his glasses.

"Dr. Collins, what is your job?"

"My job, sir?"

"You have a job, don't you? You get a paycheck, don't you?"

"Yes, sir."

"Well, what do you do?"

"I'm a second-year orthopedic resident at the Mayo Clinic."

"Do you want to be a third-year resident someday, Dr. Collins?"

"Yes, sir."

"What is an orthopedic resident supposed to do?"

Where was this going? "Follow orders?" I venture.

"An orthopedic resident is supposed to practice orthopedics, Doctor. He is not supposed to go around asking patients if they have ever considered the ontological implications of their fragile, mortal state."

"I didn't exactly—"

He jumps to his feet and points his finger at me. "We fix things. Do you understand that? We don't analyze things. We don't discuss things. We don't wring our hands and cry about things. *We fix them!* If somebody wants to be analyzed they can see a shrink. When they come to the Department of Orthopedics at the Mayo Clinic they want only one thing: they want to be fixed.

"Now get the hell out of here and go fix things. And I better not get any more reports of touchy-wouchy, hand-holding sessions in this department."

I wondered how my colleagues dealt with this issue. I suspected they did as I did: they tried to ignore everything but "the fixing." But isn't even the least perceptive of us eventually bound to question what he is doing?

What we were attempting to fix was, as BJ said, "our fragile, mortal state." But mortality can't be fixed. We can rod a femur or plate a radius, but sooner or later we have to confront the absurdity of what we do.

But, of course, BJ was right when he said what we understand doesn't matter. All that matters is what we do. No one cares how philosophically perceptive their surgeon is. They just want someone to fix them. There would be time for "all that philosophical crap" later. But that philosophical crap doesn't go away. It's still waiting for you when you get back to your call room late at night.

I discussed this once with Jack Manning. Jack never seemed interested in delving into the deeper meaning of his work. He was content to fix what he could, and let it go at that. When I told him what was bothering me, he very accurately articulated the problem surgeons face, and then succinctly enunciated the appropriate response to it.

"Shit happens," he said with a shrug. And then, looking up, "Fuck shit."

It was 4:30 I had to make rounds in an hour and a half. I didn't even bother to kick off my shoes. I lay down, shifted the stethoscope in my hip pocket so it wouldn't dig into my side, and pulled up the blanket from the foot of the bed.

"Fuck shit," I said, and closed my eyes.

# CHAPTER TWENTY-ONE

*January*

We were slouched in chairs in a second-floor classroom of the Medical Sciences Building listening to one of the research fellows drone on about biomechanics. Behind me I heard a chair scrape and someone softly sigh. I looked out the window and watched the branches of a snow-clad elm rise and fall in the cold north wind. Next to me Bill Chapin was drawing an anatomically correct picture of a naked woman.

I leaned over and pointed at the picture. "What kind of vector force makes them stick out like that?" I whispered.

"These," he said, blowing off the erasure debris and holding up the picture for scrutiny, "are yet another example of the beauty and symmetry of nature."

In front of the class Dr. Hai Wong was discoursing earnestly about an esoteric biomechanical principle known as the Right Hand Rule.

"Many orthopedic residents never master the concept of the Right Hand Rule. This is very sad." He frowned and stuck out his lower lip to be sure we understood the concept of sadness. "The Right Hand Rule is very important. It appears on the Orthopedic Board Exam every year. If you don't know the Right Hand Rule, you will flunk the Board Exam. You will remain a resident for four more years, living on macaroni and cheese." He nodded slowly to impress upon us the terrible culinary fate that lay in store for those who did not master the concept of the Right Hand Rule.

I looked out the window again. It was a beautiful day for skiing. I was imagining myself schussing effortlessly down a long hill of powder. My eyes drifted closed and my head began to sink forward on my chest.

"Dr. Collins!" Wong said sharply.

My head snapped up.

"Explain the summation of forces in the Right Hand Rule."

I realized that I was being asked to provide enough rope for the good doctor to hang me. I obliged by mumbling something about perpendicular forces in a three-dimensional construct.

Dr. Wong's eyes bulged and he began drumming his fingertips together in front of his lips. "Dr. Collins," he said, "are you particularly fond of macaroni and cheese?"


We were into the third week of our Basic Science rotation, a six-month classroom stint during which we studied histology, biomechanics, immunology, and other nonclinical disciplines. During this period we were relieved of all patient-care responsibilities—no call, no beeper, no clinics.

The six months of Basic Science marked the dividing line between junior and senior residency. When we finished Basic Science we would be senior residents. It was a time for study, but there was plenty of time for relaxation, too. It was like going back to college.

Some of us had no problem slipping back into a college mentality. Frank Wales innocently asked Dr. Wong one day if he knew how to "make a hormone." Dr. Wong patiently replied that not all hormones were amenable to re-creation in the laboratory setting. Frank shook his head sadly and said that was "a gol-dern shame," and that he "surely would like to see someone up there in front of the whole class trying to make a hormone."

It was with some misgivings I had started Basic Science. I looked forward to a relaxing six months, but I had no interest in histology and biomechanics and immunology. I knew they were important disciplines. I knew that histologists and biochemists and immunologists were the ones who would someday cure cancer and eradicate disease. I respected and admired them. I just didn't want to be one of them.

From the day I started medical school I knew I was meant to be a clinician, not a researcher. Basic Science, with all the academic grunt work, was just one more boring hurdle I had to jump before I could get on with the real business of medicine: seeing and treating patients.

But I also realized that these six months of Basic Science would give me the opportunity to catch up with my peers. Even though I had closed the gap considerably, I still felt behind everyone else. Basic Science would be my chance to draw even.

When our last class ended at 4:30, we shuffled out of the Medical Sciences Building, notebooks under our arms. The sun had already set but there was still enough light to see heavy clouds drifting in from the west. It looked like more snow was on the way.

"Who wants to get a brew?" Jack asked.

Bill shook his head. "I was thinking about heading over to the Rec Center to play some handball."

Jack turned to me. "Mike?"

"Not me. I'm moonlighting in Mankato tonight. In fact," I said, looking at my watch, "I have to get moving. I'm on at six."

"With that car of yours you'll be lucky to get there by 6:00 A.M."

"There's nothing wrong with my car."

"Yeah," Bill said, jumping in to defend me. "Just because it has no brakes, no shocks, no muffler, and is hitting on five of eight cylinders doesn't mean something's wrong with it. It's a car with character, a car for the ages."

"Yeah, the Dark Ages," Jack said. "Anyway, the hell with his car. Do you want to get a beer or not?"

"Decisions, decisions. I don't know whether to play handball or drink beer."

"The bars don't close for another ten hours," I said. "Why don't you do both?"

They looked at each other. "For a guy dumb enough to drive ninety miles in a death trap, that boy is all right," Jack said.

"I'll stop at home, pick up my gym clothes, and meet you at the Rec Center in half an hour. Now, *you,*" Bill said, turning to me, "better get a move on. At this very moment, just outside the town of Mankato, there is a drunken, infected, child-molesting, workman's comp, biker dude who's got his Harley cruisin' at about ninety. He is all set to crash head-on into a four-hundred-ton semi. This gentleman is going to require your tender ministrations shortly." He smiled. "Good luck, Doctor. With that car of yours, you'll need it."

I said good-bye to Bill and Jack and trotted out to the parking lot. I tossed the biomechanics notebook on the front seat of my car. As I swung out of the lot, I popped the top of a can of Coke and headed west. The roads were clear, my gas tank was full, and I had an hour and twenty minutes to do the ninety miles to Mankato.

# CHAPTER TWENTY-TWO

*March*

I moonlighted every chance I got during my Basic Science rotation. I hoped to pay off all our bills and even put away a little for the future. I moonlighted so often that I could almost do the ninety-mile drive in my sleep. Sometimes I think I did.

Although I moonlighted because I needed the money, I was starting to realize how much valuable experience I gained while moonlighting. I reduced fractures, drained infections, repaired tendon lacerations. Even the nonorthopedic things I did, things like caring for heart attacks and treating ear infections, honed my diagnostic skills and made me a better surgeon.

Some weekends at St. Joe's could be relatively quiet, but this weekend I was earning every cent they paid me. I had been working for thirty-four hours and had just two more to go. I had gotten three hours of sleep Friday night and managed another hour the next afternoon. But Saturday night had been a nonstop succession of the ill, the injured, and the intoxicated.

The guy with the chest pain had finally been admitted to the CCU. The college kid with the broken hand from the bar fight had been casted and sent home. I was just finishing the prescription for the baby with the ear infection.

"Give him one teaspoonful three times a day," I said, handing the mother the prescription. "We've given him his first dose here, so you can wait 'til morning to fill the prescription." The mother nodded, folded the prescription, and put it in her purse.

"Did you ever have an ear infection when you were a kid?" I asked her.

"No," she said, shaking her head wearily, "never did."

"Me neither. But every adult who ever had one says it is the most painful thing they can ever remember."

We both looked at the baby who, thank God, had finally fallen asleep. Being careful not to wake him, I ran my index finger up and down his chubby, little forearm, feeling the baby-soft skin.

"The ampicillin will fight the infection," I said, gazing at the sleeping infant, "but it doesn't do much for the pain. Be sure to give him some Tylenol if he seems to need it."

She nodded in understanding and gave me a quiet smile of thanks. She lifted the baby to her shoulder and in a moment they were gone.

I was just about to go to bed when Johnny called back to say Helen Youngberg was here again. Helen was a thirty-seven-year-old woman with multiple sclerosis. She was a regular at St. Joe's ER. Her parents brought her in at least once a week with one problem or another. Although Helen's MS was worsening, she ignored her neurologist's advice to stay in a wheelchair; consequently, she fell a lot.

Helen had suffered the ravages of MS for fifteen years. She could barely walk, and because of optic neuritis she could barely see. Connie Fritz, one of the ER nurses, had known Helen for years. Connie told me she thought Helen was deteriorating mentally as well.

When her husband had left her five years before, Helen moved in with her parents who were in their seventies. Her ex-husband remarried, moved to Seattle, and had nothing to do with Helen. "As soon as the going got rough the son of a bitch took off," her father had told me.

Helen's parents were tough old Swedes. They never complained, but it was becoming obvious they were having a hard time caring for Helen. Helen, however, adamantly refused to consider a nursing home or long-term care facility. She kept insisting she was fine at home.

Johnny pushed Helen, who was in a wheelchair, back to us. Helen was holding her wrist. Her parents, heads hanging, shuffled slowly behind.

"She fell again, Doc," her father said. "We've told her a thousand times to call us if she has to go to the bathroom but she got up by herself. Looks like she broke her arm."

"Hi, Helen," I said. She didn't answer. Even though I had seen her several times before, Helen appeared not to recognize me. Her wrist was swollen and angulated. "I'm afraid your wrist is broken," I told her. "We'll get some X-rays, and then I'll try to put the bones back in position."

She was back from X-ray in fifteen minutes. The films confirmed a displaced fracture of the distal radius. I explained to Helen and her parents that I would have to reduce and cast the fracture. I scrubbed her wrist, then injected some local anesthetic into the fracture area. This would help but it never eliminated all the pain. Helen gasped as I mashed the bone back in position.

When I finished applying the cast I told Connie to get some post-reduction films. While we were waiting, Helen's father asked if he could talk to me. We stepped into the empty waiting room. "Doc," he said, "do you think you could keep Helen here for a day or two?" He rubbed a hand across his forehead. "I can't bring her home. My poor wife is wore out trying to look after her."

A wrist fracture is not sufficient grounds to admit a patient to the hospital. But I couldn't bring myself to tell him that. The poor man looked terrible. He was seventy going on a hundred. I knew I could admit her if I made up some bullshit about neurovascular compromise or something.

"Let me see what I can do," I told him.

I went back to Connie and told her we were going to admit Helen.

"For a wrist fracture? They'll never let you admit her for that."

"Yes, they will. Tell the supervisor she is being admitted for observation of her neurovascular status. She may need surgery."

Connie looked at me like I was nuts. I put my hand on her forearm. "Connie," I said, "we can't send her home." I pointed at Helen's parents who were slumped against each other in chairs along the far wall. "Look at them. They've done what they can. It's time to find another solution."

Connie nodded. She called the nursing supervisor to make arrangements for the admission.

The front desk was quiet except for the occasional, disinterested voice coming across the police radio. I signed a couple charts, then dictated a history and physical. There was no sense going to bed since Helen would be back from X-ray in a few minutes. I thought I'd take a quick break. I slipped on my lab coat, waved to Johnny at the front desk, pushed open the door, and stepped into the night.

I hopped over the snowbank at the edge of the sidewalk and walked thirty or forty steps until I was away from the bright lights over the door to the emergency room. It was quiet out there. I leaned against a tree and looked to the west where the moon, almost full, was just setting. The Minnesota River was several blocks away, and although I couldn't see it, on a quiet night like that one I could hear the faint, sibilant rush of its waters.

It was cold, so I clutched my thin, white lab coat a little tighter about me. I felt guilty that I had lied to get Helen admitted—and yet I felt it was the right thing to do. Helen could hardly walk, could hardly see, and was growing demented. She needed more than her parents could provide. I didn't blame Helen for trying to hang on to every possible thread of normality. I knew she thought if she went to a nursing home she would never come out. But I felt sorry for her parents, too. They were seventy years old and trying to do the impossible.

I looked back at the hospital, thinking how far away it seemed, and how far removed I was from the mortal lessons being played out within its walls. But as I basked in my invulnerability, I began to feel vaguely troubled. There was something about Helen that struck a chord in me, something more than the usual empathy a doctor feels for his patient.

I didn't know why. One could hardly have picked two more different people. I was a young, healthy, active man. She was a sick, decaying woman. But despite our differences, I could understand her frustration and anger at what was happening to her.

As I stood there watching the long shadows of the moon stretch across the open field next to the hospital it occurred to me that maybe Helen and I had more in common than it seemed. Wasn't I held just as firmly in the inexorable grasp of mortality? I didn't want to admit it, but maybe that's why I felt Helen's situation so keenly. Maybe I found her story tragic merely because it was a distillation of my own. Maybe my empathy for her was just a disguised grieving for myself.

Behind me a faint smudge of gray streaked the sky behind the leafless trees. It would be dawn soon. I massaged the back of my neck, pushed away from the tree, and brushed the dirt from the sleeve of my lab coat. I took one last, lingering look into the night and headed back to the ER.

# CHAPTER TWENTY-THREE

*April*

Her name was Julie and she had gone through a windshield.
She looked about nineteen, but it was hard to tell with all the blood. I watched as they unloaded her from the ambulance. The paramedics told me Julie's boyfriend, who was driving, had missed a curve and driven off the road a mile this side of Janesville. Julie, who was sitting next to him, hadn't bothered with a seat belt. She'd been hurled, face first, through the windshield. They found her on the side of the road fifty feet from the car. Her boyfriend, passed out, was slumped over the steering wheel, unharmed.

Julie's face was a mess. Her nose was broken. One of her ears was half-off. A large flap of skin had been torn back from her forehead. From under the edge of the partially retracted flap I could see the glittering white frontal bone.

I closed my eyes and groaned. It was 2:14 A.M. I had been moonlighting at St. Joe's for the last nineteen hours. I had been hoping to catch a little sleep, but it was going to take the rest of the night to put all this back together.

I examined Julie carefully. I could smell the alcohol on her breath, but she was conscious and oriented. Her vitals were stable. Her spine, her belly, her chest, all seemed okay. For a kid who had just gone through a windshield she looked pretty good.

Julie's mother arrived a few minutes later. I could hear her screaming at Johnny at the reception desk. "Where is my daughter? Where is she? I want to see her right now!"

Julie was down at X-ray. I figured I'd better go out and talk to Mom.

"Mrs. Arndt? Hi, I'm Dr. Collins."

She gave my hand a brief shake. "I want to see my daughter. What happened to her? How is she?"

"She's been in a car accident, Mrs. Arndt. She's conscious. She can move her arms and legs. She appears stable, but we aren't taking anything for granted. She's down at X-ray right now. She has a broken nose and some lacerations."

Mrs. Arndt took a step closer and got right in my face. "What kind of lacerations?"

"She has some pretty bad cuts on her left ear and face."

She put her hand to her mouth and staggered back. "Her face? Oh, God. Not her face."

Maybe she misunderstood me. "Mrs. Arndt, I think your daughter is going to be okay. I don't think she has suffered any life-threatening injuries."

"Her face. Oh, God, no. This can't be happening."

*Lady, did you hear what I said? All right, so she cut her face. Would you rather she was paraplegic or had a leg amputated? For Chrissake she went through a windshield. She's lucky to be alive.*

"Mrs. Arndt," I said, "as soon as the X-rays and lab tests are back I'll let you know."

"Her face," she kept repeating. "Her face."


A week earlier I had been studying in the Mayo Medical Library. I spent a lot of time there during this six-month Basic Science rotation. I had been reading journal articles on intramedullary rodding of femur fractures when I noticed that someone had left a book on the table. As I pushed it aside I glanced at the title: *Plastic Surgery of the Face* by Sir Harold Gillies.

Oh, great, I thought, a book about fat, wrinkly socialites who want face-lifts and nose jobs. This was a book I wanted to hate. Before I opened the cover I was heaping scorn on the author and the patients.

I was not prepared for what I found.

The author was a World War I military surgeon who had treated hundreds of young soldiers with disfiguring facial wounds. On the basis of all the terrible injuries he treated, he became the world's foremost expert on facial reconstruction.

The book was full of pictures. I gazed in awe at page after page of men with their noses shot away, their eyes blown out, their faces torn off. Men with bullet holes through their cheeks, with faces burned and scarred beyond recognition, with great gaping holes where their eyes or mouths should have been.

Gillies spent his career reconstructing the faces of those poor soldiers. Their hideous wounds awoke in me a profound respect for the men and the sacrifices they had made. I also felt a grudging admiration for Gillies himself. He was not what I had expected. I had always considered cosmetic surgeons little more than glorified beauticians fawning and fussing over trivial matters of appearance.

But now, in Mankato a week later, I realized that's what I was about to do—fawn and fuss over a trivial matter of appearance. Why wouldn't I just run some 2-0 silk and close her laceration in ten minutes? So what if she was left with a horrible scar? What's wrong with a scar? It isn't painful. It doesn't interfere with the ability to see, to eat, to breathe. It has absolutely no functional significance.

Appearance. That's all I was doing, fussing over appearance. Then why did I have this feeling that what I was about to do was terribly important, that it was imperative to make her face as close to "normal" as possible?

As I went on with my preparations, I noticed there were more nurses hovering around than usual. It took me a moment to realize why. They didn't want this young girl to have a terrible scar. They wanted me to know I had to do a good job.

And I did know it. I was having a hard time explaining it to myself on a rational basis, but I knew it. I knew a hideous scar would change Julie's life, would change it a whole lot more than mis-setting a radius fracture would. Mis-setting a radius fracture would cripple her arm. Leaving her with a hideous facial scar would cripple her life. I could acknowledge the reality of that statement, but I pretended not to understand it.

I had always scorned patients who wanted their wrinkles smoothed or their noses reshaped. What a waste of time and energy, I thought. Those people should worry about more important things. They had a lamentable preoccupation with appearance.

But now I was beginning to wonder. If appearance doesn't matter, then why not leave the baby with a cleft lip alone? Why not let her grow up with a deformed face and then tell her that looks are not important and that she has a lamentable preoccupation with appearance? And why not tell Dr. Gillies to leave the disfigured face of the soldier alone, too? Why not tell the soldier to shut up and quit complaining?

What I seemed to be saying was that babies with cleft lips and soldiers with burned faces deserve cosmetic surgery, but middle-aged socialites with double chins do not. But who was I to impose my value system on middle-aged socialites? Who was I to say they should accept what they have and stop whining? What if one of them got in a car crash and smashed her facial bones to smithereens? Would I still say she should not have cosmetic surgery? What if it was Patti who was in the car crash—would I want her to go through life with a disfigured face?

I wanted to be consistent. I wanted to say that it wouldn't matter to me if Patti's face was horribly disfigured. I would still love her. Her essence, her inner self, would not have changed. Why would rearranging a few folds of dermis, or changing the relationship of the maxilla to the mandible matter to me—or to her?

If I truly loved her, loved the essence of her, I shouldn't care about the outward shell. She was still my wife, my soul mate, despite whatever happened to her zygomatic arch. Why would it matter to me if she had two less, or more, skin folds on her cheek? Didn't, shouldn't, love transcend such things?

But this was all silly sophistry and I knew it. Appearance matters. Never mind why. It matters.

Julie's blood tests and X-rays were back in fifteen minutes. Everything was normal. When I finished reading the X-rays I went to talk to her mother.

"Mrs. Arndt, Julie's X-rays look good. She has a broken nose, but her spine and skull films look good. All her blood tests are good, too. It appears that she has no serious internal injuries."

"Can I see her?"

Oh, boy. This was going to be touchy. If I didn't let her in, she would probably go bonkers. But if I did let her in, she was likely to flip out when she saw Julie's face.

"Mrs. Arndt, she's pretty bloody. Are you sure you want to see her?"

"Yes. I want to see my daughter."

I led her back to the trauma area. "Just for a moment," I said. "I still have to repair the lacerations and that's going to take quite a while." I pulled back the curtain where Connie was just giving Julie a tetanus shot.

"Oh, my baby, my baby," Mrs. Arndt said, wringing her hands in front of her. Connie had dressed the forehead and ear with a gauze wrap, but blood was soaking through.

"I'm okay, Mom. I'm okay."

Her mother stared at her from the foot of the cart, tears streaming down her face. "Oh, my poor baby," she said. "Thank God you're okay." She took Julie's hand in both of hers and kissed it. "Are you in much pain, sweetheart?"

"My head hurts," Julie said, "and my ear."

"I'd like to see her cuts," the mother said to me.

"Mrs. Arndt, I don't think—"

"I am her mother and I want to see them."

I nodded to Connie who began unraveling the gauze wrap from Julie's head. The ear, which had been held in place by the gauze, flipped over and hung upside down. On Julie's forehead a large clot of blood slid from under the partially retracted flap.

Mrs. Arndt gasped and covered her mouth with her left hand. "Oh, God," she said, grabbing the IV pole for support. Connie came around from the other side of the cart and took her by the arm. "This way, Mrs. Arndt," she said, leading her to the waiting room.

"Julie," I said, when her mother was gone, "your X-rays and tests turned out fine. It looks like your only injuries are the cuts on your face and your ear, and a broken nose."

I slipped on a pair of gloves and dabbed at her forehead with a 4x4. I dropped the red, soggy mess in the kick bucket next to me and then inspected her cuts. She had a large flap that extended from the middle of her hairline down and into the left eyebrow, then back up and into the left temporal region. The ear was almost avulsed, being attached by a one-inch stretch of skin inferiorly.

I positioned her head on the cart, extending it a little to expose the laceration. Fortunately for Julie, even though there were small pieces of dirt and glass scattered throughout the wound, the edges of the laceration were fairly sharp.

"Is it going to hurt?" Julie asked from under the sterile drape.

"Only a little when I stick you with the needle for the numbing medicine."

She was silent as I drew up the lidocaine. "How bad is the cut?" she asked.

Thank God she hadn't seen herself in a mirror. She would have freaked out if she saw that flap of skin hanging from her forehead.

"Well, Julie," I said as I began injecting the lidocaine around the periphery of the laceration, "it's a pretty long gash, but I think I'll be able to repair it pretty well."

"Will I have a scar?"

Will she have a scar? Jesus Christ, she went through a windshield. She's lucky she has a head. Does she think this huge gash is going to heal back like magic with no scar? Maybe I should have shown her what it looked like when she came in.

"Yes, Julie, there will be a scar. But I am going to do everything I can to make it as small as possible."

"Oh." She started to cry.

"I'm sorry, Julie. But still, you should be grateful. You went through a windshield tonight. Things could have been a lot worse."

She was shaking with sobs now.

"Julie, honey," Connie told her, "you have to hold still now so the doctor can sew you up." She reached under the drape and took Julie's hand. "You want him to do a good job, don't you?"

"Mmm-hmm," Julie sniffled.

"Okay, then, hold real still. If anything hurts you, tell Dr. Collins and he'll numb you up a little more, okay?"

"Mmm-kay."

I put in a couple stay sutures and began marking the skin with the sterile marker, mapping out the repair.

It's a metaphor, isn't it? I thought in a moment of clarity. The face, the scar, the repair. They're metaphors. There's something else, something deeper, something that explains all this irrational concern.

But that's as far as I got. The repair demanded too much concentration for me to speculate on just what that "something deeper" might be. And of course my old friend, pragmatism, wanted none of it. What did it matter? I had a job to do. Screw the philosophizing and get those first few subcutaneous sutures in.

Two and a half hours later I put in the last suture. It was 5:30 A.M. The facial repair had gone well, but I was a little worried about the vascularity of the ear. Well, we'd just have to see.

Julie's blood alcohol was .07—not legally drunk but enough to have made her sleep for the last two hours. It made things a lot easier for me, but God how I hated that alcohol breath. I felt as if I had spent half my life stitching up faces of people with boozy breath. Connie squeezed some Neosporin on a sterile tongue depressor and I applied it to the suture line.

"It looks really good, Mike," she said.

"Yeah," I said, "it came together nicely." I twisted my head back and forth, stretching my neck muscles. My neck was killing me, partly from the tension and concentration, and partly from leaning over Julie's face for the last two hours.

I whipped the drape off her face. She still didn't wake up.

"Julie?"

"Hmmm?"

"Julie, wake up. We're all done."

"Huh? Where's Martin?"

Who? I looked at Connie for help.

"The boyfriend," she whispered.

"Martin's gone home," I said. Gone to jail, rather. The cops charged him with DUI. "Your mom's here, though."

"Mmmm."

As I prepared to wrap her head in gauze I studied the repair. I had to admit, it looked pretty good. But there would still be a scar. I wondered if Julie or her mother would be satisfied.

It's a metaphor, I thought. Someday I'm going to figure out what it all means. But not now. Now I'm going to bed.

# CHAPTER TWENTY-FOUR

*May*

At five to seven on a warm spring evening I swung the old Ponch into the parking lot of St. Joe's hospital and shut off the engine. The car lurched twice, gave several consumptive coughs, and was still.

The ER was empty, thank God. I had been doing an awful lot of moonlighting while I was on Basic Science, and was praying for a quiet night for a change. I said hello to the nurses who were sitting at the desk listening to the radio. Mary was folding towels and Jenny was doing a crossword puzzle. No, I didn't know a seven-letter word for a wet-nurse. And, no, they didn't know what the cafeteria was serving for dinner.

I tossed my shaving kit on the bed in the call room and sprinted down the hall. I had two minutes before the cafeteria closed. A guy in a white apron was just closing the door as I got there. I squeezed by him, grabbed a tray, and glanced at the chalkboard at the start of the serving line.

"What the heck is Cheese Florentine?" I asked the woman behind the counter.

She shrugged and pointed her serving spoon at a steaming tray of amorphous green material. "Cheese Florentine," she said.

I still had no idea what it was, but my only other choice was lutefisk, so I took the Cheese Florentine. I ate the salad, the roll, the cherry pie, and the lemon square first. I was about to begin a cautious dissection of the warm pile of biochemicals on my plate, deciding where to make the first incision, when I heard the call for a code in the emergency room.

I dropped my fork and ran to the ER. A crowd of nurses, technicians, and red-jacketed ambulance attendants were gathered around a cart in the back corner of the ER, the spot reserved for critically injured patients. I pushed my way through the crowd and saw the motionless body of a little boy of about five lying on the cart. My crew of three ER nurses was doing all the right things: getting an IV in, starting oxygen, taking vitals.

"What have you got?" I asked Jenny as I scanned the child for injuries.

"Five-year-old boy, riding his bike. Hit by a drunk. He's been here about a minute. Mary's getting his pressure."

The kid's head was swollen to twice its normal size. The jagged shaft of the radius was sticking through the skin of the left forearm. He had a partially caved-in chest. I couldn't feel a pulse. The boy was bleeding from his mouth, his chest, his leg, his arm, and his ear.

Mary pulled off her stethoscope and shook her head. "No pressure," she said.

I opened one of his eyes and looked at his pupils. Fixed and dilated. For a moment all activity ceased. Everyone—Mary, Jenny, even the EMT doing CPR—stopped and looked at me. It was my call. Every bit of my medical training told me I should quit right there. It was hopeless. I looked at the others. They all waited, poised in mid-task.

Perhaps it was hopeless, but some things are just too terrible to accept. I pointed at the EMT. "Resume CPR," I told him. I would not let this child be taken from us without a fight.

Jenny had started an IV. I ordered steroids and mannitol for the head injury. Being careful not to extend his neck, I slipped in an ET tube. I moved around the cart, barking orders. I did a cut-down and put in a CVP. I stimulated his heart with epinephrine. I put in a chest tube. I drew blood gases from the femoral artery.

I tried to focus on my job. I tried not to listen to the drunk who was crying and slobbering in self-pity two cubicles away from us. "All of a sudden he was juss there," the man moaned. "He wasn't, and then he was, and I couldn't stop. I tried but I couldn't. Oh, Jesus, I couldn't. I juss wanna never happen . . ."

I kept feeling for a pulse, kept glancing at the cardiac monitor looking for a rhythm. Mary, doing the chest compressions, was starting to breathe heavier, gasping a little, as she counted out each compression: "One and, two and, three and, four and, one and . . ."

Still nothing. The IVs were running wide open. I couldn't think of any more meds to give. I started wondering what the hell I was doing. Why was I poking and pushing and pumping and cutting and jabbing this innocent little boy's body? Whom was I helping?

I kept telling myself that as long as we kept trying, there was hope. The little boy was not officially dead until we, until I, stopped coding him. I couldn't stop. He was just a poor kid riding his bike. He didn't deserve to die. I could not accept what was happening.

"One and, two and, three and . . ." He is not going to die.
*He is already dead.*
"Another amp of epi." I will keep going until I have tried everything.
*You already have.*
"Why aren't those gases back yet?" The family is depending on me.
*What you're doing isn't helping the family or anyone else.*

After almost an hour, when the nurses could hardly keep up with the chest compressions, when all the drugs that could be used had been used, when I could no longer pretend there was hope, I told them to stop.

The paramedics and the techs sighed and turned away. Even the janitors and the secretaries who had been standing in the background silently drifted away. The nurses stopped for a moment to catch their breath, then methodically began the cleanup.

We tried not to look at each other. We began to pay particular attention to the minute details of our job: Mary was carefully wiping down the side rails of the cart. Jenny, a clipboard in her hand, was doing inventory on the drugs we had used. I picked out a bloodstain on my lab coat and devoted ten minutes to scrubbing that one stain (while ignoring the other twenty).

We became very delicate about handling the child's body. We, who had been cutting and sticking and jabbing him for the last hour, were now careful, almost reverential with him. I lifted a hand that had been dangling from the side of the cart and placed it over his little crushed chest. Jenny took a wet washcloth and wiped the trickle of blood from the corner of his mouth, then carefully brushed the hair from his forehead. Mary gently tugged the bloody sheet from under him and replaced it with a fresh one. We did what we could to prepare him. His parents who had been clinging to each other, terror-stricken, in the waiting room, would want to see him.

There is a rule in most hospitals that forbids anyone from removing the tubes or lines that have been inserted during resuscitative attempts. They are supposed to be removed only by the pathologist or the coroner or God-knows-who. It is a rule I have always despised, and I was not going to obey it now. I was not going to let the parents see their little boy with all those things sticking out of him.

I pulled the ET tube, the subclavian line, and the chest tube. I asked Jenny to pull the IV. His skin was cooling, thickening. He wasn't bleeding much anymore. He was quickly changing from a little boy to a dead body. The end of the radius was still sticking through the skin of his left forearm. I tucked the arm under the sheet.

The nurses were wiping blood off the instruments, the cart, the floor. They whisked away the bloody debris overflowing from the garbage, all the while taking surreptitious glances at me, wondering. They knew what came next. They knew I couldn't in all mercy delay any longer.

I kept twisting the lap sponge in my hands. Those parents had entrusted their child to me. They were farmers or drugstore clerks or factory workers, and I was the fair-haired boy from Mayo, the one who was supposed to save their son. Instead I was about to tell them I hadn't saved a goddamn thing. Their son was dead.

I still have a job to do, I told myself. I will not give in. My responsibility to the dead is over, but I still have responsibilities to the living. I will not give in. I turned away from the nurses and looked up at the ceiling.

Oh, God, I thought. Oh, God.

I longed to let go, but I didn't have that luxury. I didn't get paid to let go. The others could vent their emotions, but not me. I was supposed to be there for others, not for myself. I needed to shut up and do what I could for those who were left behind.

I don't know what I said to the parents. I scarcely remember the conversation. I believe they took it well, whatever that means. I remained quite composed. I wonder if they thought I was a cold fish.

I spent the next two hours treating the patients who had been waiting with their earaches, stomach pains, and wrist fractures. It was a small emergency room so everyone knew what had happened. They were apologetic, as if recognizing that their problems paled in comparison to what they had just witnessed.

They had been listening through the drawn curtain as the drama unfolded. They heard us wage our frantic, and ultimately futile, fight; and doubtless they, too, suffered when they heard the log nurse declare flatly, "8:27 P.M. Resuscitation halted."

I must have looked more distraught than I realized. All the patients tried to encourage me. I can't recall if I was embarrassed by their efforts or if I welcomed them. Perhaps I resented them.

I left the drunk, the one who had killed the little boy, until last. He had gashed his cheek when he fell getting out of his car. Two stern-faced Mankato policemen were standing next to his cart, waiting to take him away as soon as I finished. As I stood over him, preparing to suture his laceration, I tried hard to hate him. I wanted an object at which I could direct my wrath.

"Oh, Doctor, what have I done?" he said to me. "I'm sorry. I'm so sorry."

He was so remorseful, so devastated, that I couldn't find it in me to hate him. The two Mankato cops, however, didn't have that problem. "Thanks, Doc," one of them said when I put in the last stitch. "Now this bastard is going to jail and I hope he rots there." The prospect of his rotting in jail seemed to please them. It did nothing for me. Why do we always think our pain will be less if we can make others suffer more?

At length I caught up with the rest of the work in the ER. Then I started to fill out the ER record and the accident report. I was about halfway through when I realized I couldn't remember all his injuries. Was his facial laceration four inches or six? Was it his third finger or his fourth that was dislocated?

The body was in the hospital morgue awaiting transport to the coroner's office. I had never been to the morgue before. Jenny had to tell me where it was. I went down to the basement, to the end of a long corridor. I pushed open the door and startled an owlish-looking man who must have been a pathologist. He wore thick, dark-rimmed glasses that made his eyes look huge.

"106.8 centimeters," he was saying.

The little boy's body was lying naked on a metallic table in the center of the room. The man was obviously performing the postmortem. He held a Dictaphone in his left hand, a tape measure in his right.

I introduced myself. We said a few words and then went about our business. I examined the boy and scribbled a few notes on the index card I carried in my shirt pocket. Lying pale and naked on that table, he didn't look like a little boy anymore. He looked like a dead body.

The pathologist adjusted his glasses and went on with his dictation. "Severe cranial contusion involving the right temporoparietal region . . ."

This was too much for me. Yeah, life had to go on, and, yeah, autopsy reports had to be dictated—but right there? Right then? Did we have to be in such a hurry to reduce him from a child to a report? It was hideous.

I wanted to scream at the pathologist: *Is that all you have to say? That he was 106.8 centimeters long and had cranial contusions? That's a summing up?* He was trying to reduce this little child to impersonal facts dribbled dispassionately into a Dictaphone. I wanted to choke him. *What the hell do you know? This little boy cannot be summed up so tidily. His height and the summation of his injuries don't begin to describe him.*

I was approaching the end of my Basic Science rotation, the end of my junior residency, and I was beginning to understand that there was more to that little boy, more to all of us, than can be measured with a ruler or weighed with a scale—a lot more.

If not, I thought, everything I do is pointless.

# CHAPTER TWENTY-FIVE

*June*

June had been a gift. After a cold, rainy Memorial Day weekend, a succession of warm, sunny days stretched lazily to the end of June. But June was drawing to a close, and with it, our six months of Basic Science.

Basic Science had been great. I loved the practical training: the vascular repairs we did on dogs, and the course on internal fixation of fractures. I had spent hours in self-directed study of almost every aspect of orthopedics. But I didn't spend a lot of time on the esoteric stuff: the biomechanics and histology. I had grown tired of lectures and formulae and pompous academics with inflated egos. I loved orthopedics. I loved taking care of patients. Now that Basic Science was ending, I couldn't wait to put on my scrubs and be a surgeon again.

I had gained a tremendous amount of experience during those six months. I had done so much moonlighting, had seen so many fractures and dislocations and lacerations and infections, had done so many repairs and reductions and castings, that instead of feeling inferior to my peers, as I had for the first two years, I actually felt that now I had seen more and done more than they had.

.    .    .

The trees were swaying gently in the breeze as we sat in the second-floor classroom of the Medical Sciences Building one last time. I was looking out the window watching two cardinals flirt with each other in the elm tree just outside the window.

At the end of the row Dr. Wong waited impatiently. "Dr. Collins, the exam is finished. Pass your test to me." I folded my biomechanics final exam booklet and passed it down to him. When he had collected all the exams he turned to the class and said, "All of you are to remain seated. Dr. Burke wants to talk to you."

"Aw, Christ," Bill Chapin muttered, pushing back in his chair. "What does that Irish asshole want now?"

"Hey, watch the ethnic slurs," I said.

"Yeah," Jack said, "don't forget Collins is an Irish asshole, too."

Bill, Frank, Jack, and I had a tee time at Maple Valley at one o'clock. We weren't happy about waiting. BJ stormed in ten minutes later. He wasn't happy either. He said we hadn't applied ourselves. He said we treated Basic Science like a vacation. He said medical students knew more biomechanics than we did.

"Do you think that's funny, Chapman?" He took pleasure in calling Bill the wrong name.

"No, sir."

"Then why are you laughing?"

"I wasn't laughing, sir. It's just that most medical students can't even spell biomechanics."

I winced. Bill never learned. Why didn't he just take his medicine, shut up, and let BJ move on to harassing other people? Instead Bill always baited him and invited more disaster.

"Chapman," BJ said, leafing through the papers in front of him until he found the one he wanted, "your scores in histopathology and biome-chanics are pitiful. A medical student with scores like this would never even get a residency. Did you study at all, or did you spend the whole six months goofing off?"

"I—"

"If you want to stay in this program, Chapman, you better shape up."

"Yes, sir," he said. He put his right hand behind his back and stuck up his middle finger.

"As for the rest of you," BJ said, "your days as junior residents are over. Tomorrow you will begin your senior residency. You will have junior residents working under you. You will be given a tremendous amount of responsibility, and I expect professional behavior from every one of you. This is the Mayo Clinic and every patient is to be given the best care of anyplace on this planet."

He bent his head and peered at us over the top of his glasses. "I will be keeping a close eye on this group," he said, "a very close eye." He picked up his papers and left the room.

"Keep a close eye on my ass," Bill muttered.

After BJ's pep talk, the four of us piled into Jack's Buick. We couldn't get everyone's clubs in the trunk so Frank and I, in the backseat, held Frank's clubs across our laps. We were running late, but Bill insisted we stop for a bucket of Kentucky Fried Chicken and a couple cases of Grain Belt.

"We'll stick 'em in the back of our carts," he said.

We made it to Maple Valley with four minutes to spare. Artie, the owner, was waiting for us. "I was getting worried," he said. "You guys are never late for a tee time."

"One has one's priorities," Jack told him.

"We'd have been here sooner, but we got delayed by some lunatic who wanted to talk about force couples and vectors," Bill said.

"Well, you're on the tee, fellas," Artie said as he took our money. "And you better get a move on. We got another foursome going off right behind you."

"Naked cheerleaders?" Jack asked.

"You guys watch too many movies. This is Minnesota. People here don't even get naked when they take a bath."

On the first tee Bill broke open the Grain Belt and handed us each a can.

"Gentlemen," he said, raising his beer, "our revels now are ended. Tomorrow we reenter the world of surgery. But first we'll have one last adventure. This afternoon, here at beautiful Maple Valley Country Club, we will be competing for"—he paused, eyeing each of us seriously—"the Golf Championship of the Western Hemisphere."

"Chapman," Frank said, going into his BJ Burke imitation, "your swing and your short game are pitiful. Medical students know more about golf than you do. Did you play golf at all this quarter or did you spend the entire six months looking at the pictures in your biomechanics book?"

"Wales," Bill said, "I am going to give you a stroke a hole and will still beat you to a bloody pulp."

And he did. Bill cruised in with a seventy-eight. He was one under on the front nine: three birdies and two bogeys. However, the cooler of beer and the bucket of chicken caught up with him on the back nine. He claimed the chicken made his fingers greasy. He limped in with a forty-three—still enough to beat me by four strokes.

When the round was over, when the last chicken bone had been buried in the last sand trap, when the last beer can had been tossed in the back of the cart, Jack said we couldn't just go home.

"One last beer," he said. "Tomorrow we put away our notebooks, pick up our beepers, and become surgeons again. Tonight we'll have one last beer together."

We squeezed into his car and headed back to town. Jack parked a half block down from Tinkler's, leaving the front right wheel of the Buick up on the curb.

"Well," he said when we were inside, "it's been a hell of a six months."

Jack was right. It had been a hell of a six months. I had (barely) mastered the Right Hand Rule, had learned to recognize Ewing's sarcoma under a microscope, had memorized the modulus of elasticity of stainless steel, and had written a paper on femoral shaft fractures. But more important, on my own, I had studied every aspect of orthopedic surgery I could get my hands on. I read about ankle fractures and hip replacements, ligament repairs and knee fusions, foot amputations and tendon transfers. For the first time I felt if not like a real orthopedic surgeon, then like a real orthopedic resident—and I was ready to go back to work and prove it.

But it hadn't been all work. During those six months I had also managed to get my handicap down to a twelve, and to spend countless hours reading Hemingway, Yeats, Woolf, Flann O'Brien, Neil Gunn, Shakespeare, Wordsworth, Matthew Arnold, and, I'm not ashamed to admit it, Louis L'Amour. Frank Wales was the guy who got us hooked on Louis. There were so many Louis L'Amour paperbacks in the ortho call room at St. Mary's that we had begun referring to Louis as the Patron Saint of Orthopods.

Besides golf and reading, I also had moonlighted enough times to actually open a savings account. And, in between everything else, Patti and I had managed to conceive another child.

"What is this, Birth-O-Rama?" Jack asked when he heard the news. "There is a way to prevent that, you know."

"There is?" I said. "I guess I should have paid more attention on my OB/GYN rotation in med school."


Sharon, one of Tinkler's younger, more well-endowed waitresses, had just brought us another pitcher of beer. Bill was making her listen to the story of his round of golf. "So there I am on the eighteenth hole," he was saying. "My caddy, a broken-down booze hound named BJ Burke—" He turned to her. "Ever heard of him?"

Sharon, who was studying her fingernails, shook her head. "Ah, no," she said. "No, I haven't."

"Well, never mind. He's some bum from the state mental hospital who caddied for me. Anyway, I'm about 180 out and the idiot hands me a nine-iron. A nine-iron! Can you believe it?"

Sharon shrugged. "Sounds dreadful."

"Damn right it was. But I took that nine-iron, closed it down a little, and nailed that sucker. Hit it stiff. Six inches from the pin."

"How nice," Sharon said, glancing at her watch.

"Yeah," Bill said, puffing out his chest. "Yeah, I was thinking of quitting this doctor gig and going on the pro tour."

"A couple more beers," Jack said to Sharon, "and he may run for pope."

"Shut up, Manning," Bill said. "Any guy who just finished six months of Basic Science and still can't break a hundred should be ashamed of himself. You're a disgrace to this residency."

Jack hung his head and put a hand over his eyes. "I'm ashamed," he said. "I feel so cheap, so dirty."

Sharon rolled her eyes. "Anything else I can get for you gentlemen?" she asked, trying to back away.

"Yes," Bill said. "Yes, there is." He put his right hand over his heart. "We can't go on like this, you and I, pretending we don't care for each other. Take me," he said. "Take all of me."

Jack nodded. "Yeah, Sharon, except for the gas problem and the snoring, he's really quite a catch."

"Let me get your check," Sharon said.

"Oh, good," Patti said as I came in the back door, "I was worried you were going to miss dinner. What took you so long?"

"Another rough day at work," I said, giving her a kiss.

"Phew! You don't usually come home from work smelling like that."

"Well," I said, "after we finished our biomechanics final we played golf."

"Where, in a brewery?"

"Well, you know how Jack and Frank and Bill are. They said we had to stop at Tinkler's on the way home."

"Oh, those big bullies dragged my little Mikie into a bar and poured beer down his throat."

"Something like that."

"Well, sit down. I'm glad you're home."

When dinner was over, and the dishes were done, I put the girls in their pajamas, said their prayers with them, and tucked them in bed. As I closed the bedroom door, the house was quiet. Patti was curled up on the couch listening to Carole King on the stereo. I slid her feet over and sat next to her.

"How are you feeling, hon?" I asked as I slipped an arm around her.

"Better."

"Is the baby still kicking a lot?"

"He sure is an active little thing. He's always poking me right here." She pointed to a spot low on the left side.

"Well, at least you've got Eileen and Mary Kate to do the housework for you."

"While I lie around taking bubble baths and eating bonbons."

"You know," I said, "in my next life I want to come back as a resident's wife."

She sat up, folded her hands, and looked at the ceiling. "Oh, please, God, *please* grant this fool's wish."

We laughed. I pulled her head against me and began running my hand through her hair. "You have the nicest hair," I said, burying my face in it. We sat like that for several minutes.

"Well, hon," I said finally, "tomorrow I go back to the real world—this time as a senior resident."

She sighed. "And I get to be a widow again."

I had spent a lot of time with Patti and the kids the past six months. We ate dinner together almost every night. We took the kids to the petting zoo at Oxbow Park, and to the pool at Silver Lake. We took them on long walks at Mayowood, telling them stories about their grandfathers during the war, and their foremothers during the Chicago Fire and the Potato Famine. The girls taught me how to play *Round and Round the Garden* and *Creep Mousie.* I taught them how to play *Something's Coming for Your Armpit.*

It had been a wonderful six months, but Patti knew I was anxious to get back to work. She asked whose service I had been assigned to.

"Bill Kramer's."

"Is that good?"

"Well, Bill's new on staff, so there won't be a lot of action on his service, but they never assign the new senior residents to one of the busier services like Romero, or Hale, or Cuv."

"Well, that's good," she said, looking up at me. "At least you'll be home once in a while, right?"

I couldn't wait to begin my senior residency, but at that moment, sitting with my arms around Patti, I found myself wishing I were home all the time.

# YEAR THREE

# CHAPTER TWENTY-SIX

*August*

Sarah Berenson was the girl I swore I would never forget. She was young, she was beautiful, and she was going to die if we couldn't help her.

I met Sarah during my second month on Bill Kramer's service. Bill was the youngest of the three orthopedic oncologists at Mayo. I had been leery about working with him. I was nervous not only about being a senior resident, but also about working in oncology. Oncology was the antithesis of orthopedics. In ortho, we generally dealt with healthy people and solvable problems. People came to us with torn cartilages—we removed them and they were better. People came to us with broken legs—we set them and they were better. People came to us with arthritic hips—we replaced them and they were better. I loved orthopedics. I loved going to work each day and fixing things. I loved the incredible feeling of accomplishment in what we did.

But oncology is a different story. Oncology means cancer, and cancer usually wins. Pity the poor oncologist, I thought, losing many more battles than she wins; no grateful patients thanking her every day, no tangible results affirming her competence, no happy endings. A lifetime spent signing death certificates, not op reports. Oncologists, I concluded, were better people, stronger people, than I. They did their job, they treated their patients, but they reaped none of the adulation we orthopods took for granted.


Sarah was an eighteen-year-old girl with osteogenic sarcoma of the left ilium. She had been referred to Mayo by her family doctor in Los Angeles. He told Sarah she had "a growth," it might be bad, and she needed to go to the Mayo Clinic "right away." We were left to tell her it was indeed bad, and that her only hope was a radical operation called a hemipelvectomy, in which we would remove not only the entire leg, but half the pelvis as well. Even with this mutilating surgery, Sarah's chances of survival were not good.

Sarah was a vibrant, beautiful, young woman with a perfectly proportioned body, and eyes that radiated innocence and trust. This is the Mayo Clinic, her eyes said. You will cure me. Before we had done a thing her eyes were thanking us.

Part of me liked being thanked by this beautiful young woman. It was an acknowledgment of our power, our skill. But I was uncomfortable, too. Her thanks, her trust, placed upon us a burden I wasn't sure we could shoulder. This was my first rotation as a senior resident and I was still naive enough to want to fight every bad guy, and to win every fight—but I knew the statistics, too. Sarah had osteogenic sarcoma of the ilium. The five-year survival rate was less than five percent.

But I wouldn't listen to the voice that tried to reason with me. I preferred to listen to Sarah's voice telling me how wonderful I was. I envisioned her arms around me, her wet tears on my neck as she thanked me for saving her life.

I was attracted to Sarah—but in a way I found hard to define. I wanted to be everything to her. I wanted to be her brother, her doctor, her lover—but mostly I wanted to cure her. I wanted to say, "We're going to beat this thing, Sarah, you and me." (Well, mostly me. I was going to beat it for her. It was to be my gift to her.) Cancer was the big bully forcing itself on this beautiful, virginal creature, and I was the guy who was going to stop it. We were going to drop the gloves and go at it. "Let's go, shit head. Right now. You want Sarah? Well, you'll have to come through me first."

Yeah, right. After cancer had beaten me to a pulp a dozen times in a row I would learn to keep my emotional mouth shut.

I went to Sarah's room the night before surgery. I didn't usually do that, and I didn't attempt to explain to myself why I did it that night. Five percent five-year survival, I was telling myself. That's five percent, not zero percent. That means some people make it. Sarah has to be one of those people.

It was after ten by the time I got to her room. Her parents had already left. Sarah was lying in bed, her blond hair splayed across the pillow. Her eyes lit up as I entered the room.

I started to smile, then looked away. I flipped through her chart for several seconds, then closed it. I looked at Sarah, then opened the chart once again and pretended to read something. Finally I laid the chart down and asked Sarah how she was feeling.

"Okay," she replied.

I went through the usual pre-op instructions. I told Sarah she should not eat or drink anything after midnight. I reminded her that the orderly would come for her at six o'clock the next morning. Then I asked if she had any questions. Sarah seemed confused. She seemed not to know what she was supposed to say. She shook her head and said she had no questions.

I noticed a little card in front of her and asked what it was. She showed it to me. In a neat, feminine script she had written the word "hemipelvectomy." I remembered her asking me earlier in the day what the name of her operation was and I noticed her copying it down.

"It's not in the dictionary," she said. "I looked."

No, I didn't suppose it would be.

"Can you tell me again what it means?"

I wasn't sure how to explain it to her. It had been easier to hide behind the technical terminology. It was easier to obscure the truth than to illuminate it.

I tried to act casual, as though I were asked about hemipelvectomies all the time. *"Hemi,"* I began, "is from the Greek. It means half. *Ectomy* means to remove something. So hemipelvectomy means to remove half the pelvis."

Sarah frowned in confusion. "But I thought you were going to remove . . . my leg."

"Well, we are, Sarah. Your pelvis *and* your leg."

"Oh."

We were silent for a few moments.

"Will it hurt much?" she asked.

"You won't feel a thing during the operation since you'll be asleep." I spoke with the casual ease of an experienced surgeon. "But most patients do have some pain afterward."

*Shut up, you asshole,* I screamed at myself. *You've never even seen a hemipelvectomy.*

I just stood there, squeezing her chart until I couldn't stand it any longer. I turned and started to walk away, then turned back. "Sarah," I said finally, "I . . . Well, I'll do everything I can for you."

She looked at me and smiled kindly. Now it was she who was providing the care. She was a mother comforting her little boy. She reached out, touched my forearm, and said simply, "I know you will. Thank you." She was so confident, so trusting. This was the Mayo Clinic. We would save her.

I wondered later who was more naive, Sarah or me. But, of course, it was no sin for Sarah to be naive . . .


Sarah was the first case, so the orderly came for her at 6:00 A.M. Her parents followed behind. I was waiting for them when they arrived at the surgical holding area. At the door the orderly stopped so Sarah could kiss her parents good-bye. Her father leaned forward and kissed Sarah on the cheek. He squeezed her shoulder, then quickly turned away, hiding his face from her. Her mother stepped forward, her eyes filled with tears. Sarah struggled to sit up. They tried to embrace, but the IV kept getting in the way.

"I love you, Sarah," her mother said.

"I love you, too, Mom."

They continued to reach for each other as the orderly pushed Sarah through the double doors into the brightly lit holding area. Sarah's mom kept her arm extended toward her daughter as the doors swung shut with a gasp of compressed air.

I helped the orderly wheel Sarah into the corner where I introduced her to another orderly, Luella, who was going to do the prep. While the pre-op nurse was attaching a bag of antibiotic solution to the IV, Luella explained that she was going to scrub and shave Sarah's leg. I sat at the desk as Luella swung the curtains around Sarah's cart.

I could hear Luella tear open the surgical scrub sponge and begin the prep. "I even have to get up around your private area, honey," Luella said. "Can you raise your bottom a little?" I could see the shadow on the curtain as Luella had Sarah bend her knees and spread her legs. Every bit of her pubic hair had to be shaved away.

Five minutes later Luella asked Sarah if she had ever had a catheter.

"No," Sarah replied in a barely audible voice.

"The catheter goes into your bladder," Luella told her. "That way whenever you need to pee it will just come out through the tube."

Sarah was told to spread her legs again. Luella washed her with a warm, soapy solution, then painted her with betadine.

"This might hurt a little," Luella said.

Sarah gave a brief gasp.

"There, now," Luella said. "All done. Let me get a blanket from the warmer." Luella was back in a few seconds. She tucked a warm blanket under Sarah's chin, then tore back the curtain. "Bye, honey," she said, patting Sarah on the shoulder. "Anything else I could get for you?"

"No," Sarah whispered.

An anesthesiologist came in and talked to her about the procedure. He said once she was asleep he was going to put a breathing tube in her mouth. He also said she might be given some blood during the surgery. He asked if she had any questions.

Sarah, who seemed not to have heard a thing he said, answered, "No." She lay quietly, watching the nurses scurrying back and forth between patients, starting IVs, hanging antibiotics, taking blood pressures and temperatures.

Finally I went over to her. "Sarah, have you had anything to eat or drink since midnight?" I asked.

She shook her head. "No," she said.

"Okay then, Sarah, it's time to go."

I unlocked the cart and swung it out from the stall. We passed through a series of double doors before finally entering the OR. As always, it was cold, and intensely lit. As we entered, I pulled up the mask that had been hanging below my chin. I docked the cart next to the narrow, black operating table and asked her to "scoot over." The circulating nurse whisked Sarah's blanket away and Sarah gasped at the cold. As she started to move to the OR table her gown rode up to the top of her thigh. Sarah had been told not to wear panties and she blushed as she tried to tug her gown back down. One of the nurses helped her, then covered her with a warm blanket.

Two arm boards were swung out from the side of the table and Sarah lay with her arms extended to either side. The anesthesiologist wrapped a blood pressure cuff around her right arm while one of the nurses adjusted the IV in her left. Another nurse returned with two more blankets from the warmer. Sarah tried to shrink beneath them.

Just as she was starting to warm up, the anesthesiologist pulled the blankets away and calmly mentioned he had to "place some leads." Sarah blushed again as he reached under her gown and placed several cold, sticky patches above and below her breasts. As soon as he replaced the blanket another nurse said in a cheerful voice, "Cold, sticky pad!" She slapped a large, cold pad on Sarah's right thigh. A clear electrical wire ran from the pad to a machine next to the table. "That's your grounding pad," the nurse said. Sarah smiled and nodded as if she knew what a grounding pad was.

I could see Sarah's eyes begin to glaze over. "I have just given you a little something in your IV to relax you," the anesthesiologist said. I stood next to her, leaned over. "Are you cold, Sarah?" I asked as I tucked the warm blanket under her chin.

"Please," she said, her voice raspy and small. Her eyes welled up with tears. She struggled to sit up. "Please don't . . ."

As the anesthesia began to take effect she sank back down and closed her eyes. "Don't worry, Sarah," I said. "We'll take good care of you."

The anesthesiologist told Sarah to take a couple big, deep breaths . . .

From start to finish it was a horrible operation. Oh, nothing went wrong from a technical sense, but the whole thing was so wrong, so unfair. For the first time I began to wonder if we were part of Sarah's problem rather than part of her salvation. Even the prep and drape seemed obscene. We turned Sarah on her right side, and prepped her from the low back to the knee. We then covered everything except her left leg with sterile drapes. Sarah had now disappeared, buried under a mound of blue drapes. We were no longer operating on a person. We were operating on a tumorous appendage emerging from a blue hole.

Bill took the sterile marking pen and outlined his incision. I held Sarah's leg high in the air and watched in awe as the purple line skirted her labia, swung up almost to the lower abdomen and then dipped back and around the upper buttock. When he had finished he dropped the marking pen on the Mayo stand and held out his hand.

"Scalpel."

It was a long, bloody operation. I was constantly clamping and cauterizing and placing retractors, trying to give Bill the best exposure. As the operation progressed, Bill and the anesthesiologist conversed frequently, deciding when to give the next unit of blood or fresh frozen plasma. There was a steady flow of blood products going in her arm and oozing out her surgical wound.

Every move we made caused more bleeding. Blood pumped and oozed and leaked and squirted. We soon became oblivious to it. Our gloves became tacky and thick with it. Blood spread up our sleeves and coated the front of our gowns. Blood seeped into the surgical sheets and spread down the side of the drapes. Blood dripped on our shoes and soaked into the blankets the nurses had cast on the floor in front of us.

Slowly, over several hours we began to separate Sarah's long, shapely leg from the rest of her body. The two edges of the incision grew farther and farther apart. When we finally severed the iliac bone, the leg dangled obscenely from a few posterior tendons. These Bill quickly severed and the leg was free.

I lifted the leg, the gaping wound at the top still oozing blood, and slid it into a sterile, plastic bag the circulating nurse held for me. As the leg dropped into the bag the nurse couldn't hold it and it fell to the floor. One of the other nurses came forward and helped wrap the leg. I glanced briefly over my shoulder as the circulator, carrying her burden in front of her, exited the room and headed to Surgical Path.

Bill and I still had another couple hours of work to do. There was a question of how many sacral nerves we could spare. If we took too few, we would increase the chance of tumor recurrence. If we took too many, Sarah's bladder and perhaps her anal sphincter wouldn't work.

I stared into her huge open wound and saw virtually nothing familiar. It was all virgin territory to me. I had assisted on plenty of hip operations, but had never seen the inside of the pelvis like this.

That must be the vaginal wall over there, I thought. And up there, the side of the bladder; behind the bladder, a portion of the rectum and the sacral plexus. And dangling everywhere were the tangled shreds of nerves, vessels, and tendons.

Closure seemed to take forever. There were several layers of tissue that had to be approximated. Then we had to decide how best to close the skin. Should we trim here? Advance there? Tuck this? Excise that?

By the time we placed the last drain and put in the last suture, it was early afternoon. Sarah's pressure was stable. She had been given eighteen units of blood but had come through the procedure well.

Bill went to talk to the family, and left me to apply the dressings. I peeled away the bloodstained sheets. For a brief moment, after the drapes had been removed and before the nurses had been able to cover her with a fresh gown, Sarah lay totally exposed.

We tried not to stare. All of us—myself, the anesthesiologists, the nurses—quickly found other things for our eyes to do. But the truth was there now, the truth we had tried to hide under all those layers of sterile, blue surgical drapes. Sarah had no leg. There was a long line of black sutures across the left side of her lower abdomen, and below that—nothing.

I applied the dressings, being careful not to disturb the catheter. Sarah's skin was pale and cold. I lifted the drain reservoirs onto her belly, then we moved her off the operating table and back onto the cart. It wasn't difficult; she didn't weigh much anymore. The nurses covered her with warm blankets, and then I wheeled her to the recovery room.

Sarah's post-op course was stormy. She ran a fever for four days. The inferior portion of her wound dehisced. Her labia swelled so much she couldn't urinate. I tried to put a catheter back in her, but she was so swollen I couldn't find the urethra. Finally we had to call a urologist to do it.

But Sarah was a marvel. She kept thanking us for all we were doing, and apologizing "for being such a bother." She was as bright and engaging as ever. I couldn't understand it. I thought if I lost my leg I would be inconsolable. I would never laugh again. Like Job's wife's I would want to curse God and die.

I longed to ask Sarah about it, but I didn't know how. What would I say, "Sarah, shouldn't you be more upset about having your leg chopped off?" Finally I approached Annie Cheevers, Sarah's nurse. Annie had become like Sarah's big sister.

"Sure, we talk about it," Annie told me. "And *of course* she's sad about losing her leg, but she says it's made her realize how many things she *hasn't* lost. She says it's like a millionaire who loses a thousand dollars—he's sad, but he's still not that bad off."

I thanked Annie and nodded thoughtfully, as though I understood, but I still didn't get it. I was still too ignorant about what a scalpel could, and could not, do. All I could see was that we had taken away her leg. I didn't yet understand that there are some things no surgeon, no disease, can ever take away.

Annie and the other nurses adored Sarah. The day nurse would come back at night to sit and watch TV with her. The night nurse would stay in the morning to have breakfast with her. The PM shift nurse would call as soon as she got home to be sure she was given her midnight meds. And how they guarded her. Every order, every procedure, was scrutinized.

"Dr. Collins, she just had her hemoglobin checked yesterday. Can't we wait until tomorrow to check it again?"

"Dr. Collins, I noticed a little serous drainage coming from the bottom of her incision."

"Dr. Collins, don't go in now. She just fell asleep. Couldn't you come back later?"

How thrilled we were three days after surgery when Sarah stood and took a few tentative steps on her crutches. She was pale and trembling as she looked at us for encouragement.

And how shocked I was seven days after surgery when I knocked on her door and heard Annie Cheever's voice tell me to "wait just a minute." I stood at the door, looking at the curtain that had been drawn around the bed, thinking Sarah must be on the bedpan. But why the bedpan? She had been walking to the bathroom for several days now. Finally Annie pulled back the curtain, gestured dramatically at Sarah, and said, "Ta-da!"

Sarah was sitting on the edge of the bed smiling at me. Annie had helped her wash and set her hair and apply her makeup. She was stunning. I stared at her, a myriad of emotions swirling inside me.

Annie began to laugh. "I think he likes it, Sarah."

"Sarah," I said, "you look . . . nice." It was my turn to blush.

Annie was outraged. "Nice? That's all you can say? That she looks nice?"

"I, uh, well you look *really* nice. I mean—"

They both laughed. They knew they had succeeded.

Sarah went home a few days later. She gave me a big hug and thanked me for saving her. I looked away and said nothing. I saw her two weeks later when she returned to Rochester for a post-op visit. After that I moved to another service. But for months afterward I would see the black suture line running across the stump of Sarah's left pelvis; and I would wonder just what it was Sarah thought she hadn't lost.

But I was busy with other things, other patients, and soon I stopped thinking of Sarah at all.

# CHAPTER TWENTY-SEVEN

*October*

On September 29 I left Bill Kramer's orthopedic oncology service and was assigned to adult reconstructive surgery with Dr. Frank Satterfield. I had learned a lot from Bill, but I was happy to get away from cancer and get back to hip replacements and fractures.

I had been on Frank Satterfield's service for three weeks. We were just finishing Mr. Schaeffer's total hip surgery. Frank stepped back, snapped off his gloves, and told me to close.

"Nice job today, Mike," he said. "I think you're ready. The next one is yours."

The next one was mine.

I had never done a total hip replacement before. I had been assisting on them for two years now. Attendings had let me do parts of the procedure, but I had never done the whole thing myself. Being the assistant had become routine, almost boring, and I had been yearning for the chance to do it all.

But now that my time had come I was scared stiff. Total hip replacement was a complex, almost daunting procedure. The incision had to be in just the right place, then the fascia had to be incised, and the abductor muscles released—just enough, but not too much. Then the capsulotomy, and the osteotomy of the femoral neck at precisely the right distance above the lesser trochanter. Then the reaming of the acetabulum and the proper positioning of the cup. Then the reaming of the femoral canal, and the choosing of the correct stem size and length. Then the cementing, and the placing of the femoral prosthesis in just the correct amount of anteversion. Then the selecting of neck length, and finally the closure, being sure to get the capsule closed and the abductors repaired and the fascia approximated. And if everything was done correctly, if the approach and the implant selection and the cementing and the orientation and the repair were all done just right—you would have a happy patient with a painless hip.

But there were pitfalls everywhere. Damage the sciatic nerve, and the patient could be partially paralyzed. Mal-orient the components, and the hip could dislocate. Cut the femoral artery, and the patient could bleed to death. Over-ream the acetabulum, and you could break through the wall of the pelvis. Impact the stem too vigorously, and you could fracture the femur. Kink the femoral vein, and the patient could die of a pulmonary embolus. Repair the abductors improperly, and the patient could limp for the rest of his life. Rush the cementing, and the prosthesis could loosen prematurely. Take too long with the cementing, and the patient could go hypotensive and die on the table. Break your sterile technique, and the hip could get infected. Fail to evaluate the medical condition, and the patient could die of a heart attack. Give the wrong anesthetic, and the patient could become a vegetable.

And all the time you are doing this, you are living with the realization that a mistake could ruin your career. Screw up once, blow some big operation, and no attending in his right mind would ever let you operate again.

You get your chance. The attending hands you the ball. If you run with it, if you do a good job, then you are on your way, your reputation is made. But if you drop the ball, if you screw up with your first chance, there might never be a second one.

"See one. Do one. Teach one." That was the way we jokingly described the learning process when I was at the Veterans Administration Hospital in medical school. But this was the Mayo Clinic and residents were very heavily scrutinized before they were allowed to operate. I was being given my chance, and I wasn't going to blow it.

I checked with Amy, Dr. Satterfield's secretary. She told me our next total hip was scheduled for the following Monday. That would give me the weekend to go over the procedure, step by step, being sure I had it all down.

I pulled the X-rays for the case and templated them, planning which size prostheses I would use. I poured over Campbell's *Operative Orthopedics,* and Charnley's *Low Friction Arthroplasty of the Hip.* I went over all the pertinent articles in the *Journal of Bone and Joint Surgery.* I reviewed the anatomy in Hollinshead's *Anatomy for Surgeons.* I even called Jack Manning who had gotten to do his first total hip the quarter before.

"Try not to cement the femoral component upside down," Jack told me.

"You're a big help."

"Relax, Mike. You've probably scrubbed on a hundred hips. You've done parts of this operation plenty of times. The only difference is this time you're going to do them all. Hell, I watched you do that subtroch fracture last month. You looked like you had been doing them your whole life. Those are a hell of a lot harder cases than total hips."

On Monday morning I was at the hospital early. I finished rounds in time to go over my notes on the surgical technique one more time. The hip replacement was our first case. Steve DeBurke, the junior resident, helped me get the patient prepped and draped. Then we sent word to Dr. Satterfield in the surgeons' lounge that we were ready. While Frank scrubbed in, I got the marking pen and outlined the incision. This was my subtle way of reminding him that he had promised this case to me.

When he was gowned and gloved, he approached the operative field and said to me, "You ready?"

"Yes, sir."

"Then let's go," he said, gesturing at the patient. "We're wasting time."

Once I was into the case I was surprised at how smoothly it all went. I had the operation down cold, and was too focused to be nervous. When the femoral component had been cemented and the hip reduced, Frank stepped back from the table. He had hardly said a word the entire case but

I was glad he had been there. It was reassuring to know he could help if I ran into any problems.

"Pretty damn good job," he said to me.

"Thanks, Dr. Satterfield," I said.

He shucked off his surgical gown and said, "I'll be in Room Four doing the knee scope. You guys finish up in here and get the next one going."

When he had gone I finished repairing the abductors and the capsule, then turned to Steve. "You know what this means, don't you?" I said, stepping back and motioning to him to assume the head surgeon's position.

Steve's eyes lit up and I could tell behind his mask he was grinning like a little kid. "I was hoping you wouldn't forget," he said.

There was an unwritten rule among the residents that if the senior resident got to do the case, the junior resident got to do the closure. I had watched Steve assist, and though he was a little too raw to do the abductor repair, I was sure he could handle the rest of the closure. Of course it took him ten minutes longer than it would have taken me, but he had fun doing it and I had fun helping him.

And when we had finished the day, when we had changed out of our scrubs and into our street clothes, and completed afternoon rounds, I realized something was different. I was no longer just a student. That's what residents are, in a sense, students. They are still learning. Well, I had done a total hip that day—by myself. And I could plate an ankle, scope a knee, and fix a both-bone forearm fracture, too. Hell, in a pinch I could probably do a rotator cuff repair, although I didn't feel too sure about that.

I felt a growing confidence, a feeling that all these years of work were starting to pay off. Four years of high school, and four years of college, and four years of medical school, and a year of internship, and two years of ortho with two more to go. That's seventeen years. Sometimes it seemed like I would never be done, that I would be a student forever. But after today I knew that wasn't true, for the first time I didn't feel like a student. I felt like a surgeon.

# CHAPTER TWENTY-EIGHT

*December*

I was halfway through my third year when I realized I might have a chance to be named chief resident. The selection wouldn't be made for another few months, but I knew the last two and a half years of intense study were paying off. Instead of hiding at every conference, I found myself answering questions, even making suggestions. "Why, you're no stupider than the rest of us," Frank had said to me recently.

What made it easy was that I loved what I was doing. I loved seeing patients and I loved doing surgery. In the operating room I was becoming more comfortable. Besides having done a total hip, I had removed a torn cartilage through an arthroscope, and had released a carpal tunnel. I had rodded a femur, plated a tibia, and wired an ulna.

It was heady stuff, and I was proud of what I had achieved. But to be appointed chief resident I would have to do more than just survive the next few months. I would have to shine.

Patti went into labor with our third child, Patrick, three weeks before Christmas. She started feeling contractions one morning around six, just as I was leaving for work. She asked me to wait five minutes, then five more.

Finally, after a particularly strong contraction, she said, "I think it's time. We'd better go to the hospital now."

I paged Dr. Satterfield and told him Patti was having her baby. He told me I could take the whole day off. "Let me know if it's a boy or a girl," he said.

I bundled up the kids, took them out to the car, and got them in their car seats. Then I went back inside and helped Patti. We dropped the kids at Alice Chapin's and headed to Methodist Hospital. By seven, when she was admitted to the OB floor, Patti's contractions were four minutes apart and getting stronger. By eight she was fully dilated.

"You don't waste any time, do you?" said the nurse who wheeled her into the delivery room.

Five minutes later Bill Chapin and Frank Wales, holding surgical masks over their faces, showed up. They had been waiting to start a case down in the OR when Alice Chapin called Bill and told him Patti was in labor. They came to say hi.

"Mike," Bill said. "How ya doin'? How'd that tibial plateau fracture go yesterday?" Then, almost as an afterthought, he looked at Patti who was by then up in stirrups. "Oh, hi, Patti," he said. "You're doing fine. Just keep pushing."

Patti was well into her labor pains and couldn't care less that two of her husband's friends were watching her deliver. Patrick was born a few minutes later.

"Angry-looking little critter, isn't he?" Frank asked as he watched Patrick scream and squirm.

"Well, it's been fun," Bill said, after the baby had been cleaned and suctioned. "We gotta go. Duty calls." He turned to Kenny Billings, Patti's obstetrician, who was delivering the placenta. "Nice job, Kenny," he said. "Now don't forget the lidocaine when you sew her up."

Patti pushed herself up on her elbows. "Will you two get out of here?"

Frank looked at Bill. "I reckon she means us." He shook his head sadly. "It must be the drugs talking."

As they turned to go, Bill said, "Don't worry, Patti, we'll be by later this morning with coffee and donuts—hopefully in time for *Jeopardy.*"

"I can hardly wait."

During the next two days there was a steady stream of residents in and out of Patti's room. The nurses found it difficult to enforce the visitation rules since almost every visitor was a doctor. Patti told me at one time there were four doctors, two of their wives, the mother of one of Patti's college roommates, a nurse, and Patrick in her room at the same time. She took it all in stride. She would grab Patrick from the arms of one of the residents, throw a blanket over her chest, and "plug him in," as she called breast-feeding.

She came home on Saturday. There were so many flowers that we filled the backseat of the car with them. When we got home, Sue Manning, who had come over to watch Eileen and Mary Kate, helped me bring in the flowers. Then she kissed Patti. "Gotta run," she said. "I'll be back this afternoon." She gave me a peck on the cheek and told me Patti needed peace and quiet. "Peace," she repeated, staring intently at me. "And quiet."

What was that supposed to mean? Did she think I was going to attack Patti that afternoon?

"I thought I'd give you at least 'til tomorrow," I said to Patti later, when I told her of Sue's warning.

"It would be your last act on this earth," Patti said.

"Fine. Have it your way. You'll come crawling to me in a day or two."

She held her hands low across her abdomen. "Don't make me laugh," she pleaded.

On Monday I tried to get home as early as I could. I came in the back door about six and hung my coat on the back of a chair.

"How are you, hon?" I asked as Patti turned from the sink.

"I am so glad you're home," she said, drying her hands and giving me a hug.

"Me, too." We stood there holding each other, her head against my chest. "Where are the kids?" I asked.

"Playing in the basement."

I started to pull away, to call them.

"Don't," she said, still clinging to me. "Just let me stay here for a minute before they come up."

I laid my head on hers and stroked her hair. "Long day?" I asked.

"Long life," she said with a laugh. "When do I become the rich doctor's wife lounging at country clubs, getting my nails done, and having maids make my bed?"

"Any day now."

"Yeah, right."

Just then Eileen came into the kitchen. "Daddy's home!" she shouted. Mary Kate pounded up the stairs and the two of them ran over and hugged my leg. I bent down, kissed them both, tickled them in the armpit, and said I was glad to be home because I hadn't spanked a kid in two days.

"Where's the baby?" I said to Pat who had been wedged aside by the two little girls.

"He's asleep in the crib."

"Let's go see your brother," I told the girls.

"Yay! Yay!" they said, clapping their hands. He was their favorite toy. They liked to poke and prod and pull at him like he was one of their Barbies.

"You stay away from that baby," Patti said. "If you wake him, I'll murder all of you. The poor thing needs his rest."

*The poor thing needs his rest*—and this from a woman who had just given birth to her third baby in three years, a woman who had defied her parents to marry a guy with no money, a guy who then tore her away from home, moved her four hundred miles away, and then left her alone for days at a time.

Patti was at the sink again, her back to me. I watched as she wiped away a wisp of hair with the back of her hand. Overcome with a sudden feeling of tenderness, I came up behind her and put my arms around her.

She could tell by the way I held her something was wrong. "What's the matter?" she asked, trying to turn around and face me.

But I held her tighter and bent my head down closer to hers. "I'm what's the matter," I whispered in her ear, "and you're what's not."

"What are you talking about?" She wiggled free and turned to face me.

I smiled sheepishly and held out my arms to her. "I was just thinking that for a guy who works a hundred hours a week at two different jobs and who has a wife, three kids, and no money, I'm a pretty lucky guy."

# CHAPTER TWENTY-NINE

*January*

On January 4, the day I started as senior resident on Marty Shaw's hand service, our financial situation became even more precarious. When I went out to start the old Pontiac that morning it made a terrible grinding noise, shuddered once, and was still. I tried everything, but I couldn't get it to start. Finally I phoned Mr. Jensen at the Standard station. He grumbled that the damn thing probably died of carbon monoxide poisoning. He said with the junk heaps I drove he wasn't sure if I was studying to be a surgeon or an undertaker.

For Patti's sake he agreed to come and take a look. He checked under the hood, turned the key, and spat when he heard the groaning sound the car made. He told us to forget it. The car was dead. Totally and irrevocably dead. Brain dead. Flat line. Elvis had left the building.

"Thanks for the coffee and sweet roll, Mrs. C.," he said to Patti.

Patti smiled and thanked him for coming.

"Splurge, Doc," he told me as he climbed back in his truck. "See if you can get something with less than 150,000 miles on it this time."

When he had gone, I siphoned the gas, removed the spare tire, and called Ernie Hausfeld at the junkyard again.

"Collins. Oh, yeah. Aren't you the Mayo doctor?"

"Yep. That's me."

"You're getting to be a regular customer, Doc."

He didn't have to rub it in.

"You know the routine. You drive it in, you get thirty-five. We tow it in, it's only twenty-five."

"It's not going to start, Ernie. You'll have to come and pick it up."

"No problem. Jimmy'll be there in half an hour. Be sure you have the title ready."

Three hours later the tow truck pulled up in front. "Hey, Doc," Jimmy said as he hopped out of the cab. "Nice t'see ya again." He walked around to the back of the truck, yanked at the hitch, and slipped it under the front bumper. He leaned inside the back of the truck and pressed a button to raise the front of the car. There was a snap and the bumper fell off.

"Jesus Christ," Jimmy said. He stood there, hands on his hip, staring with disgust at the car. Then he looked at me. "So, what kind of doctor did you say you were?"

I knew where this was coming from. How could I be a real doctor when I drove nothing but clunkers that got towed to the junkyard?

"I'm a veterinary gynecologist," I told him.

"Figures."

He picked up the bumper and tossed it in the back of the truck. Then he crawled under the Ponch and secured the hitch to the frame. When he was done he stood up and slapped the dirt and snow from the seat of his pants.

"You got the title, Doc?"

I handed it to him and he reached into his shirt pocket and pulled out two tens and a five. "Here," he said. "Don't spend it all in one place."

A week later I bought an old Chevy wagon from a dairy farmer in Zumbrota. The car was another rust bucket. Someone had spray-painted it a flat gray color that made it look like a battleship. It had no muffler and the dull roar of its engine made it sound like a battleship, too.

My first stop was at Jensen's Standard station to fill it up. Blackie, Jensen's old Lab, shuffled over to lick my hand.

"Hey, Doc," Mr. Jensen said, walking out from the garage and wiping his hands on an old shammy. He looked at my car and stopped smiling. "You got a license for that boat?" he asked. He waved his hand back and forth in front of his face. "Phew. Turn the damn thing off before we all choke to death."

"So," I said, gesturing at the car with my open hand, "what do you think? Not bad, huh?"

Jensen walked slowly around the car, eyeing it with disgust.

"You're actually going to let your wife and those poor kids ride around in this damn thing?"

Apparently he didn't care that *I* was going to ride around in this damn thing. He opened the front door and looked inside. Then he turned and spat. "Fer Chrissake you can see the street right through the floor."

"Well, it's—"

"You shouldn'ta paid more than five hundred for this bucket of bolts."

"Yeah, but our other—"

"Poor Mrs. C.," he said, shaking his head sadly. "The things you do to that woman."

Like the mailman, the garbageman, the ladies at the grocery store, and every shopkeeper in Rochester, he loved Patti. They all did. And they all felt responsible for her. They all harbored the sneaking suspicion that her husband wasn't quite worthy of her (a suspicion her husband also harbored).

When I finally got the car home and showed it to Patti, she put on a brave face.

"It's, uh . . . nice," she said. "But how come it looks like that?"

"Like what?"

"That gray color. It looks like a battleship, or something."

"It's coated with a special rust preventative," I lied. "And, really, it's not bad for seven hundred bucks, don't you think?"

"It's just that . . . well, it doesn't look like a car."

It didn't sound like a car or drive like a car either. When I took it to work the following Monday, Jack Manning saw me pull into the parking lot and yelled, "Fleet's in!"

"Hey, sailor, want a good time?" someone else called.

But still, it ran. The main problem with it was neither the noise nor the appearance. It had a temperamental heater. For as long as we owned the Battleship I could never figure out why sometimes the heater worked and other times it didn't.


A week after we bought the Battleship I was scheduled to moonlight. The temperature hadn't climbed out of the single digits in ten days. As I sat on the edge of the bed trying to figure out how early I had to get up the next morning, I could hear the wind moaning through the fir tree outside our bedroom window.

It was easier to work backward.

I have to be in Mankato by seven, I thought. The roads should be plowed, so that means I can leave Rochester about 5:30. Rounds'll take an hour, so that's 4:30, plus ten minutes to drop the beeper at Bill's. That makes it about 4:15.

I never allowed time for showering, shaving, or brushing teeth. I just hoped things would be quiet when I got to Mankato so I could shower and shave there. I set the alarm, turned out the light, and snuggled in next to Patti. But before I could settle in I remembered the weather forecast.

Shit, I thought. It's supposed to be twenty below tonight. I'd better get up at two and start the car. I'm screwed if it won't start in the morning.

I rolled over, turned on the light, and reset the alarm.

At two o'clock I groaned and shut off the alarm. I sat up, rubbed a hand across my face, sighed, and pulled on a pair of sweatpants. As I shuffled toward the kitchen, I could hear Mary Kate's rattley breathing in the room next to ours. I pulled on my parka, and then stepped into the Sorrels I had left inside the back door. I didn't bother to lace them.

I opened the door and stepped into a clear, frigid night. The wind was gusting over the rooftops and rushing through the deserted backyards. I could see the skeletal frame of our swing set, legs planted deep in the crusted snow. One of the swings, its seat covered with an inch of frozen snow, was twisting in the wind. As I crunched through the snow to the garage I could feel the hairs in my nose freeze with each breath.

I heaved up the garage door, flicked on the light, and lifted the hood. I needed to take off the air filter, but the upraised hood blocked the light, and left the engine in shadows. Largely by feel, I undid the wing nut and removed the filter. I blew on my fingers and then held them under my armpits. When a little feeling came back in them, I bent over and gave the carburetor a couple flips. Finally I came around, got in the driver's seat, gave the accelerator two quick jabs, and turned the key. The starter groaned once, twice, and the car kicked into life. I held my breath. This was when the engine would sometimes quit on me. But the steady rumble continued.

I got out, replaced the air filter, slammed the hood, and scrambled back in the car. I scrunched down, head on my chest, hands under my thighs, waiting for the engine to warm up. Finally, after ten minutes, I gave it a couple revs and shut it off.

I pulled down the garage door and staggered back into the house. I tossed my coat on the chair next to the heat duct, kicked off my boots, and felt my way through the dark house to our bedroom.

I sat shivering on the edge of the bed as I reset the alarm for 4:15. I could hear Patti's slow, regular breathing from the other side of the bed. I could feel the warmth coming off her. I was so cold. If I could just slowly inch right up next to her . . .

"Oh, God!" Patti screamed. She jumped a foot off the bed.

"Sorry, hon," I murmured contritely.

"You're freezing. You are absolutely freezing. You're like an iceberg." She was flopping around, jerking covers every which way, trying to interpose as much material between our two bodies as possible.

"I was out starting the car."

"Naked?"

"No, but it's twenty below out there."

She said it felt like it was twenty below in here, and rolled away from me. I lay quietly on my side of the bed.

A minute later she relented. "All right," she whispered, "come on." She lifted the covers and I scooted over. She was on her back. I draped my right leg over her thighs and my right arm across her chest. I pressed as much of my flesh against hers as nature would allow. She gave a little gasp. "Oh, my God," she said. I felt a shiver run through her.

I lay still, listening to the branches of the fir tree scrape against our window, feeling the house tremble slightly with each gust of wind. I was safe. I was warm. I was under four covers with my hand on the warm breast of the woman I loved. I was in heaven.

"Mr. Jenin?" I said softly. It was ten after five. I had already seen the other ten patients on our service. Mr. Jenin, who had a wrist fusion the day before, was the last one. I turned on the lights. "Mr. Jenin?" I said, a little louder.

"Huh?"

"Good morning. It's Dr. Collins."

"Oh. Hi, Dr. Connolly. Is anything wrong?"

"No, sir. I just wanted to see how things are going."

He looked at the clock next to his bed. "Things?" he said hoarsely. "Going?"

I laid the chart on the chair next to his bed. He winced slightly as I peeled back the dressings from his arm. "Looks good," I said, replacing the bandages.

"Do you feel this?" I asked, running a finger along the side of his hand.

"Uh-huh."

"Can you move your fingers, like this?"

He did.

"Good. Have you had much pain since surgery?"

"Yes, but the medicine helps."

I talked to him about the physical therapy he would have later that day, apologized for waking him so early, and told him Dr. Chapin would be by to see him later that day.

It was still dark when I pulled up in front of Bill's house. It seemed every other weekend Bill, Frank, or Jack was stuck holding my beeper for me. They must have taken pity on me since they never refused. Bill had agreed to do it this time. I told him I would leave my beeper in his mailbox rather than wake him up.

God, it's cold, I thought as I trotted up the sidewalk to Bill's front door. I wonder if beepers can freeze?

I laid the beeper in the bottom of the mailbox. I also left a note thanking Bill and listing all the patients.

It must be 5:30 by now, I thought. I walked around to the front of the car so I could read my watch in the headlights. 5:36 A.M. Well, I'd have to hurry.

As I pulled away from Bill Chapin's house, the announcer on KROC said it was nineteen below. I prayed this would be one of the days when the Battleship's heater would work.

Highway 14 was deserted at that hour and I kept the Battleship cruising along at seventy. The car had no dashboard light, and since it was still dark, I occasionally had to turn on the overhead light to see how fast I was going.

The wind was streaming in through the holes in the floor. At seventy miles an hour and the temperature near twenty below, the windchill had to be approaching a couple hundred below. There was a four-day-old copy of the *Post-Bulletin* on the seat next to me. I spread it across my lap and started fiddling with the heater. I turned it off and on. I pounded my fist on the dashboard. I jiggled the control knob. But, after fifteen minutes, as I passed Mantorville, I realized there would be no heat on this trip.

I had another seventy-five miles to go. My legs were shaking and I was starting to lose feeling in my feet. In desperation I looked into the backseat. Next to the car seat I saw Mooey, Mary Kate's brown-and-white, stuffed cow. The car swerved onto the shoulder as I stretched behind me and grabbed the cow.

Poor Mooey. There would be no coming back from this mission. I wedged her into the largest hole in the floor. Immediately the cold draft up my pant leg diminished noticeably. " 'Tis a far, far better thing you do than you have ever done before," I recited.

Mooey seemed unimpressed.

When I finally got to Mankato I had a hard time getting out of the car. My knees and ankles were stiff like an old man's. I stumbled into the ER and waved a hand at the nurses. Thank God the place was empty.

"Gonna shower," I said, my teeth chattering.

After ten minutes in the shower I was finally warm enough to get out and shave. When I pushed my shaving cream dispenser, it made a guttural, groaning noise. A small wad of snow plopped from the nozzle. It was frozen solid. I tossed it back into my shaving kit and shaved with soap instead.

It was a wonderful day to be at Mankato. The high temperature was forecast to be around ten below. It was just too cold to go out, so the ER was empty for most of the day. The hospital paid me by the hour, so whether I saw a hundred people or three I made the same.

I spent most of the afternoon in the doctors' lounge watching the Canadiens play the Bruins. Every couple hours I went out and started the Battleship. I had parked it against the wall outside the ER. Around four o'clock I turned off the hockey game, went to the call room, and took a nap. An hour later the nurses called to say we had a patient, a Mankato cop with frostbitten ears. He had spent the last hour at Mt. Kato, Mankato's one and only ski hill, looking for a missing skier who turned up later in one of the local bars.

"There's not a lot we can do for this," I told the cop as I lathered ointment on the tips of his ears. "Just be sure you keep them covered so they don't get damaged any further."

When he had gone, I went to the cafeteria and had dinner. I sat alone in the corner, a plateful of pork roast, corn, mashed potatoes, and gravy in front of me. For once I was conscious of being alone. Around me, in groups of twos and threes, nurses and techs were talking and laughing. I worked away at my meal, listening to them talk about bridal showers and car problems and TV shows.

One of the nurses at the table next to me saw me laugh at a story she was telling. She flashed me a smile, letting me know that she didn't mind my listening. But I was embarrassed all the same. I finished my meal and wandered back to the call room. I lay down, took out Campbell's *Operative Orthopaedics,* and started to read about ankle arthrodeses. I was sound asleep at eight o'clock, the book lying on my chest, when the phone rang.

"We need you," Connie said. "An ambulance just called. They're on their way in with a guy in full arrest."

I grabbed my coat and sprinted down to the ER. Over the loud-speaker came the call, "Emergency room! Emergency room! Emergency room!"

Within three minutes all the ER nurses, the respiratory tech, the lab tech, and a pharmacist were waiting with me. I calmly checked the crash cart and waited for the ambulance. I had run enough codes by this time that they were becoming almost routine.

The ambulance roared into the bay with full sirens going. The driver hopped out and swung open the back doors. The paramedics were doing CPR on an obese, cyanotic-appearing man. I followed them as they wheeled the patient in.

"Fifty-one-year-old guy," the paramedic gasped between chest compressions, "chest pain for two hours . . . collapsed at home . . . his son, a high school kid, started CPR right away . . . we were there in eight minutes . . . never got a pulse."

We cut off his shirt, slapped on the cardiac leads, and started an IV. I gave him some bicarb, then epi, then more bicarb. He was in V-fib so I shocked him. I went up to his head and intubated him, went down to his groin and drew a femoral artery blood gas.

During the first few furious minutes when I was trying to do ten things at once, I looked up and saw the anguished face of a high school kid with a letter jacket standing at the foot of the cart watching the feverish activity, watching his father's cyanotic face and sightless eyes. A few seconds later someone whipped the curtain closed, and I never saw the kid again. He was the son, though. He had to be. I could see the resemblance.

I put in a central line and gave some more drugs. I tried the defibrillator again. It didn't work, any of it. After another half hour I called the code. The man was dead.

As I sat quietly at the desk, filling out the death certificate, and the ER record, I remembered the kid's eyes: the anguish and fear and confusion. How incredibly fast it must have come upon him. He sees his father clutch his chest and fall to the ground. There is a moment of confusion and panic. What is it? What has happened? Then the terrible realization that it must be a heart attack. His father needs CPR. Can he do it?

Oh, God, he thinks, why didn't I pay more attention to this stuff in health class?

He begins, clumsily. Is this the way? Is this how you do it? Then the desperate, plunging chest compressions, the awkward attempts at mouth-to-mouth, the intense longing for the ambulance to get there. Oh, God, where are they? He pushes the hair from his face and goes on. He sees his father's face growing purple, feels his lips growing cold. As he struggles on, he hears his mother's anguished sobs behind him.

Finally the paramedics arrive and he is pushed aside. He doesn't know if he did the right thing. Has he helped his father? Or has he killed him? He backs farther away, wedging himself into a corner, staring as the paramedics wage their desperate battle. Soon his father is spirited away in an ambulance. He and his mother follow in their car.

At the hospital, strangers are cutting off his father's clothes. They are sticking tubes in him, shocking him with paddles. He stands at the foot of his father's cart watching it all. He can hardly bear to watch, but he can't tear himself away. Finally someone closes the drape and he can see no more.

A few minutes later a doctor in a white coat comes out to tell his mother that her husband is dead. The doctor never speaks to him. No one does. When he thinks of his father all he can see is the bloated, purple face with that tube sticking out of it.


Two hours later, when the code was over and the death certificate filled out, when the janitors had mopped the floor and the nurses had restocked the crash cart, when the PM shift had gone home and the coroner had come to claim the body, I was still slouched in a chair at the desk. I kept going over the code in my mind, asking myself what I could have done differently. I couldn't think of a single thing. I ran a perfect code. But I kept seeing the look in the eyes of the kid with the letter jacket, and the fact that I ran a perfect code did nothing for me.

Death, suffering, failure. They were the enemy, but they didn't play by the rules. Sometimes, even when I did everything right, they still won. I couldn't give up the childish notion that things ought to be fair. When I ran a perfect code, when I did everything right, the patient ought to live. What more could be asked of me? What more could I give? Day in and day out I did the best I could, the best anyone could—and so often it wasn't enough.

It had been four hours since I had started my car. I knew I should go out and start it. I grabbed my lab coat from the back of the chair and told Connie I'd be back in a couple minutes. She told me there was a guy in Three with an infected elbow.

"Get an X-ray, a CBC, and a sed rate," I said as I left.

The ER doors slid open. As I stepped outside, every bit of warmth was sucked out of me. I groaned through gritted teeth and wrapped my lab coat around me as I opened the door of the Battleship and plopped down. I turned the key and the engine roared into life. Thank God. Within two minutes I was shivering uncontrollably. My head and shoulders were hunched forward, my arms clutched to my chest, my thighs squeezed together. My breath was condensing into a frozen mist on the inside of the windshield.

After five minutes, just as I was ready to shut off the engine, I noticed a trickle of warmth coming from the heater.

Why now? I wondered. I drove ninety miles and the damned thing never threw out a single bit of heat. Now, after sitting out in the cold for fourteen hours it decides to work. I revved the engine a couple times, shut it down, and trotted back inside.

Some questions, I realized, are never going to be answered.

# CHAPTER THIRTY

*March*

Sometimes it seemed there was so much bullshit. Patients could be rude to us and we had to take it. Attendings could abuse us and we had to take it. Silly, senseless jobs that had nothing to do with our education needed doing and we had to do them. Even though we were no longer junior residents stuck doing narc rounds and holding retractors, there was still plenty of ignominy to go around.

Boys. That's what we called ourselves—Coventry's boy or Romero's boy or Kramer's boy. We were at their beck and call. We did what they told us to do. We operated when they let us; we assisted when they didn't. Sometimes they listened to our suggestions, sometimes they ignored them. When they wanted something done they issued their commands and we just nodded our heads and said, "Yes, sir." We had to live with all the ambiguities of being thirty-year-old, highly educated men and still in positions of subservience.

Maybe that's why I liked fixing fractures so much. Fractures appealed to me in a way no other part of orthopedics did. Unlike other areas of medicine (and other areas of life), everything about fractures was straightforward. Cardiologists might bullshit about whether the patient actually had a heart attack. Neurologists might bullshit about whether the patient actually had a stroke. But with fractures, there was no way to bullshit. As soon as the X-ray was developed, everyone knew exactly what the problem was, and exactly what the solution was.

With fractures you didn't have to wait for weeks or months to see how things turned out. X-rays provided immediate, tangible documentation of our work. There was no hiding behind academic credentials, or how lousy your assistants were, or whether the night crew could find the Synthes set. The X-ray didn't care about any of that stuff. The X-ray climbed to the top of the highest hill and held itself up for all to see. And if you had done your job well, you could take pride in comparing the shattered, malaligned bones on the pre-op X-ray to the perfectly reduced, plated bones on the post-op X-ray. There was your proof. There was your honor.

Even though I was a senior resident, I still had to take call—and I was having a very busy day. I had made rounds, seen a couple consults, drained a foot abscess in the ER, and fixed a hip fracture on one of the old Franciscan nuns who had worked at St. Mary's back in the sixties. Tom Hale, the attending surgeon on call, scrubbed in on the case with me but let me do the whole thing, skin to skin.

"Nice job, Mike," he told me as we looked at the post-op X-rays. "Everything looks perfect."

Things slowed down around five o'clock, so I phoned Patti. She and the kids came over to have dinner with me in the hospital cafeteria.

"Eee-yew," Eileen said, looking at the plate of food in front of her. "What is that?"

"That's Swiss steak, honey," Patti said. "Try it. It's delicious."

"It looks like barf."

"It does not look like barf. Now be a good girl and eat it."

We were about halfway through dinner when my beeper went off.

"Dr. Collins, please call the ER, 5591, 5591, 5591. Please call the ER, 5591."

I found a phone and was back in two minutes. "It's a both-bone forearm fracture," I said. "I have to go."

Patti smiled and shrugged her shoulders—another ruined dinner. What a surprise.

I kissed Patti and the girls, rubbed Patrick on the head, and trotted down to the ER where Steve DeBurke, the junior resident on call, was waiting for me.

"Hey, Steve," I said. "What have you got?"

"Joanna Haverman, a thirty-nine-year-old lady who fell at her daughter's skating party. She's got a nasty both-bone forearm fracture."

"Open?"

"No, closed. She's got a good radial pulse but her arm's pretty crooked."

I looked at the X-rays. Steve was right. Her arm was angulated almost sixty degrees. I went in and introduced myself to Mrs. Haverman. I told her she was going to need surgery.

I went over the operation with her, describing exactly what would be done, and what the risks were. Steve had already talked to anesthesia. An OR would be ready for us in half an hour. I called Tom Hale and discussed the case with him.

"Have you done one of these before?" Tom asked.

"Yes, sir. Several times."

"Okay. Go ahead, but call me if you have any questions or problems."

While I was talking to Tom, Steve brought Mrs. Haverman up to the OR. I couldn't wait to get started. Fixing both-bone forearm fractures was one of my favorite operations.

I let Steve do the approach to the ulna. He hadn't done much surgery and was thrilled to make one of the incisions and put in a few of the screws. I did the rest of the operation myself.

I was sitting in the recovery room leaning back in a chair when Steve brought me the post-op X-rays. "Looks good," he said.

I held the X-rays up to the light. The fractures were in perfect position, the plates and screws right where they should be. I got the pre-op X-rays and put them up on the view box right next to the post-op films. The contrast between the crooked, shattered bones pre-op and the perfectly reduced and fixed bones post-op was striking. I smiled and thought how wonderful it was to do this for a living.

Steve plopped down in the chair next to me. The poor guy looked beat. I thought he could use a little encouragement.

"Nice job on the approach to the ulna," I said.

He shrugged his shoulders as if he didn't care. "Thanks."

I could see that it was getting to him—all the long hours and the endless scut work. He seemed to have lost sight of where he was headed. I didn't blame him. I remembered how I felt as a junior resident. But he also needed to learn to take comfort where and when he could. The fact that we had just done something wonderful seemed to have escaped him.

I wanted him to know how lucky he was to be able to do things like this. I took the post-op X-ray off the view box and handed it to him. "Look at this," I said. "This is what makes everything worthwhile."

Steve held the X-ray up to the light. He looked like he was still wondering what I was talking about.

"Hang in there, Steve," I said. "You won't be a junior resident all your life."

I heard the recovery-room nurse talking to Mrs. Haverman who was just waking up. I grabbed Steve by the arm. "Come here," I said. I went over and talked to Mrs. Haverman. I told her the operation went well and her bones were back in position. She moved her fingers for me and said her pain wasn't nearly as bad as it had been before surgery. She had tears in her eyes as she thanked us. I could see Steve was touched.

"Bring it on, BJ," I mumbled to myself as we were walking away.

"What?" Steve asked, frowning and leaning his ear toward me.

I laughed in embarrassment.

"I was just telling BJ Burke to bring it on—all the shit, and all the scut work, and all the abuse. To be able to do what we did tonight is worth any price. This is why I want to be a surgeon."

Steve laughed. "Bring it on," he echoed.

# CHAPTER THIRTY-ONE

*June*

I wiped my forehead with a lap sponge and said, "For a place that is so god-awful cold in the winter, it sure gets hot in the summer."

I was sitting in the empty waiting room of St. Joe's ER in Mankato. Mary and Rita, two of the nurses, were sitting with me. We were watching a rerun of *Bonanza*. We hadn't had much business all day. This was the fourth day in a row with temperatures and humidity in the nineties. It was too hot for people to go out and hurt themselves.

The hospital was rumored to be air-conditioned but no one believed it. Rita, who weighed all of ninety pounds, was fairly comfortable; but Mary, who hadn't weighed ninety pounds since she was six, was roasting. She was holding her long brown hair up over her head, and had draped an ice pack low across her neck.

"I don't get paid enough to put up with this," she panted.

It had been seventy-six degrees when I left Rochester at 5:30 that morning. A thick, steamy haze obscured the sunrise. At seventy miles an hour I kept cool enough, but I could almost feel my car slicing through the heavy air that smothered the fields and woods. As I passed Loon Lake, near Waseca, I could just barely see the figure of a solitary fisherman in a boat about thirty feet from shore lazily laying down casts on the surface of the misty lake.


About five o'clock that afternoon an ambulance called to say they were bringing in a guy with a broken nose and a cut on his forehead. Rita and I heaved ourselves out of our chairs and went to check him out. Mary wiped her forehead and said she'd be along in a minute.

Our patient arrived five minutes later. He was telling a joke to the paramedics as they wheeled him in. ". . . so then the plumber says to the guy, 'I think I can save your wife but the bishop's a goner!' Ah-ha-ha-ha!"

The paramedic at the head of the cart shook his head and cracked a smile. "We gotta go, Sal," he said, rubbing the patient's shoulder. "You take care, and go easy on the brews next time."

I motioned the paramedic over. "What've you got?" I asked him.

"The dumb shit spent the afternoon sitting in a lawn chair on his driveway. He had a cooler next to him, and his feet in one of those little, plastic baby pools. We found eighteen empty beer cans next to his chair. When he finally got up to take a leak he was so plastered he fell flat on his face. Did you see the guy's nose?"

"Yeah, I saw it. There goes his chance for the cover of *GQ*."

I said good-bye to the paramedics and went over to the cubicle where Rita was getting our patient's vitals.

"You're beautiful, baby," the guy was saying. "You should be in Hollywood not here."

Rita wasn't buying it. "Sir," she said, "please hold your arm still so I can take your blood pressure."

His forehead was wrapped with a bloody gauze bandage against which he was holding an ice bag. I removed the bandages so I could examine his injuries. He had a long laceration across his forehead, and his nose wasn't just broken, it had landed in another zip code. It was mashed way over to the left and flattened against his cheek. Dried blood rimmed his eye sockets. Apparently, however, he was feeling no pain.

"Hey, Doc, how's it goin', hah?"

"Mr., ah . . ." Dawn handed me his chart. "Mr. Pagulia. How are you, sir?"

"Listen, Doc, I gotta tell ya something." He propped himself up on his elbows and leaned forward to speak confidentially. "The ice bag them ambulance guys gimme is leaking. Looka this shit," he said, holding up the bloody, dripping bag. "It's drippin' all over me. In fact—" he paused and looked at me wide-eyed—"I think I'm getting water on the brain." He burst into laughter. "Ah, Jesus! Water on the brain!" He fell back against the cart, shaking with laughter. He jarred his head enough to make his laceration start bleeding again. "Get it, Doc?" he said between belly laughs. "Water! On the fuckin' brain!"

"An interesting observation, Mr. Pagulia. By the way, have you been drinking this afternoon?"

"What gave you that idea?" Rita whispered to me.

"Just a few beers," he said.

"A few beers." I nodded. "How many, do you think?"

"Ah, five or six maybe."

"Five or six."

"Maybe more. I dunno. Who's counting? It was hotter 'n shit out there."

"How did you hurt yourself?"

He struggled to sit back up again. "I got attacked, Doc."

"You did?" I looked over at Rita. That's not what the ambulance guys said.

"Yeah." He nodded his head, making the laceration bleed even more. "Yeah, the fucking driveway hit me right in the face! A-ha-ha-ha."

I wrapped a roll of Kerlex around his head and then sent him for nasal, skull, and C-spine films. A half hour later I could hear him down the hall as the X-ray tech was wheeling him back.

"Volare," he was singing, "wo-wo."

The tech laid the films on the counter and rolled her eyes. "He asked me to marry him," she said.

"Cantare. Wo-wo-wo-wo."

I picked up the films and was snapping them up on the view box when he called over to me. "Hey, Doc! You know 'Volare'?"

"No, sorry. I took Greek in high school not Latin."

He frowned and muttered, "What the fuck?"

"Well," I said, walking over to him, "good news. Your skull and neck films look good. The only thing broken is your nose."

"My nose? It is?" He reached a paw to his bloody face and felt his nose. "Son of a bitch. The old schnoz hung a Louie. Hey, Doc, the fuckin' thing is pointing at my ear."

"Don't worry, sir. It can be fixed."

"Shit, yeah," he said. "I've had it fixed ten times before."

Rita began assembling a suture tray for me. "6-0 nylon," I told her.

"So, Doc," my patient said when I returned, "how do you like this doctor thing?"

I replied that although it was hard work I liked this doctor thing a lot.

"Yeah," he said wistfully, "I thought of bein' a doc myself."

"Really?" I said, unfolding the edges of a sterile towel. "I'm sure you would have made a very interesting doctor."

"Fuckin'-A right," he said. He struggled to sit up and I pushed him back down.

"Sir, you have to lie still now so I can sew up the cut on your forehead."

He gave no sign that he heard me. "Yeah," he went on, nodding his head and making it impossible to drape him. "I thought a lot about bein' a doc." He lapsed into a short silence. "Medicine's great. You know, spending all day telling broads to take their clothes off for ya."

I heard Mary snickering over near the crash cart.

"Well, sir, that's not really—"

"Can you imagine," he went on, "every day, beautiful broads, completely naked, hanging all over you."

"You'll feel a little pain when I put in the numbing medicine," I said as I drew up the lidocaine. He didn't flinch. It made me wonder if he even needed a local anesthetic.

"So, what's it like, Doc? You know, being around all those naked women every day?"

Rita opened a suture for me and dropped it on my field. She cocked her head and looked at me innocently as if she, too, wanted to know.

"Mr. Pagulia," I said, "it really isn't very often we have to ask women to remove their clothes."

He smirked. "Yeah, right, Doc." This man knew a cover-up when he saw one.

"No, seriously, sir. I rarely ask my patients to disrobe."

He looked up at me. "Aren't you a real doctor?"

"Yes, sir, I am."

"Then whaddaya mean you don't tell 'em to take their clothes off?"

By now all work in the ER had ceased. Everyone was listening to our conversation. Rita, who was standing in the corner behind Mr. Pagulia, looked at me questioningly, gestured at her blouse, and started to unbutton the top button. I gave her a dirty look and told her to get me some more sterile towels.

"Sir," I said, "there is no need to have women remove their clothes for most orthopedic problems."

He wasn't sure if I was a liar or a fool who had wasted four years of medical school. "What's that got to do with having some broad get naked for ya?" His laughter came in great rolls that echoed around the ER. "I'd just tell 'em I can't tell what's wrong with their ankle until I see what their bazumbas look like."

I finally got him to lay still so I could cover his face with the sterile drape. I tried to switch the conversation to other things but his muffled voice continued to escape from under the drape constantly harking back to naked women, breasts, and pelvic exams.

In desperation I explained that most doctors, myself included, did not spend a lot of time with unclothed women. He was obviously dismayed and disillusioned. His dreams of a career in medicine were being shattered.

We then started talking about what kind of work I did. I told him about setting fractures, repairing ligaments, and replacing joints. He seemed fairly interested.

"And yer called a ortho-peedist, huh?"

"That's right," I said encouragingly.

"And you spend most of your time fixing bones and shit, huh?"

"Yes, I do."

"So you don't get no chance to check out naked broads, huh?"

I groaned. I thought we were off this subject. "No, sir, I really don't."

He thought about that a moment and then gave me a look of pity.

"Well, Doc," he said, "don't let the bastards get you down. I'm sure if you do a good job with all this bones and shit, someday you'll get your chance to be a gynecologist."

# CHAPTER THIRTY-TWO

*June*

My third year was coming to an end. In another week I would start the final year of my residency. Jack Manning had been selected chief resident for the first six months of the year, but the chief resident for the last six months had not yet been announced. There was still hope for me.

It seemed Rochester was having a special on kids with wrist fractures that summer. Every night on call I got one or two of them. Tonight it was a five-year-old kid who fell out of his bunk bed.

When the ER paged me I closed my eyes, groaned, and ran a hand across my face. Not another one! I still had one last consult to see. This was going to royally screw up my night. I told the nurses on the ortho floor that I had to see a wrist fracture, but I'd be back as soon as I could.

I trudged down to the ER, picked up the chart, and went back to examine my patient who was sitting in his father's lap, sniffling quietly. The boy was wearing Donald Duck pajamas and holding a well-worn stuffed animal that looked like Goofy. His left wrist was bent back about forty-five degrees.

Well, I thought, you don't need to be an orthopod to make this diagnosis.

I hadn't even ordered an X-ray yet, but I had already decided what was wrong, what needed to be done, and how long it would take. I was becoming very good at this sort of thing. I was becoming quite proficient at reducing fractures, repairing ligaments, injecting shoulders, and scoping knees—but something was wrong. Despite my growing competence, my work wasn't fun anymore. It was as if I had become a factory worker, mindlessly performing the work in front of me, but taking no enjoyment from it, anxious only to get it done.

But I was impatient with my self-analysis, impatient with being distracted from the job at hand. What difference does it make? I thought. I've got work to do.

I introduced myself to the father and then tried to talk to his son. I leaned over and asked him what happened but he wouldn't answer me. He wouldn't even look at me. He turned his head away, clutched his stuffed animal, and shrunk deeper in his father's arms. Fine. I gave up and called X-ray. I wasn't about to waste any more time.

Five minutes later the tech appeared. She squatted down next to the boy and stuck out her lower lip. "Oh, Danny," she said. "Did you hurt your arm, sweetheart?"

The kid looked at her and his eyes welled up with tears. He nodded his head. "I fell out of my bed."

"Oh, you poor little thing." She put her hand on his cheek. "Well I'm going to take a picture of your arm and then this nice doctor is going to fix it for you, okay?"

"Mmm-kay."

"Would you like me to take a picture of Goofy, too?"

He looked at her in amazement. Did she really mean it?

The tech continued to squat next to him, smiling encouragingly.

Danny nodded his head and handed Goofy to her.

I stood in the corner, wondering why the child would talk to an X-ray tech when he wouldn't talk to his doctor. As the tech continued talking to the boy I grew impatient. Was she going to keep jabbering to him all night long? I had a job to do, and we were wasting time. Finally the tech set up her portable machine and took the wrist films. Then she laid Goofy on a cassette and took a film of him, too.

While I waited for the X-rays to be developed, I made arrangements to take the kid to the OR. I called Bonnie Wilk, the anesthesia resident on call, and told her I would like to do it in the cast room just off the main OR. Then I called the cast tech, John "Ski" Kowalski, and asked him to meet me in the cast room in fifteen minutes.

The X-rays showed a badly displaced fracture of the distal radius and ulna. But the little kid wasn't interested in the X-rays of his wrist. He was staring at the X-ray of his stuffed animal. A faint gray silhouette of Goofy was outlined against the black of the film. While the X-ray tech and the boy took turns pointing at things on Goofy's X-ray, I explained to the parents that the bones would have to be reduced, and that the least painful way to do this was under a general anesthetic.

"I don't think I will have to make an incision," I said. "I can usually manipulate the bones back in position, then put on a cast. Danny can probably go home tonight, but let's see how things go."

We got the kid up to the cast room and then had to wait fifteen minutes for anesthesia to show up.

"Sorry," Bonnie said. "We were just finishing a C-section."

I looked at my watch and nodded impatiently. Yeah, right.

It had been a long day and I wanted to get to that last consult. And besides, when we were done, I'd have to talk to the parents again. That would take another couple minutes. I made a note to myself to be sure I remembered their name this time. The last time I fixed a fracture like this, I did a perfect job, but when I went out to talk to the parents I couldn't remember their name or their child's name, either. It had made for a very awkward conversation.

Ski, quiet and competent as usual, wheeled the cast cart over and started selecting the plaster rolls we would need. When Bonnie finally got the kid asleep she nodded to me and said I could go ahead.

"Okay, Ski," I said. "You know the drill."

I bent the elbow to ninety degrees. While Ski held the arm I applied traction to the hand, stretching the fracture. Then, while continuing to apply traction with the right hand, I increased the deformity just enough to let me wedge my left thumb under the edge of the fracture. Then I levered the dorsal edge of the distal fragment over the dorsal edge of the proximal fragment, and finally pushed the whole thing volarly. I could hear a little crunch as the bones slipped back into place.

I knew the reduction was perfect. I told myself that I had done my job. All right, I thought, so far so good. Now let's get the cast on and get junior here to the recovery room.

"Keep the elbow at ninety," I told Ski, "and be sure the wrist is in volar flexion while I put the cast on."

Ski nodded and held the arm in perfect position. As I began wrapping cast padding around the boy's arm, I noticed a blue tattoo under the edge of Ski's scrub shirt.

"Hey, Ski," I said, pointing to the tattoo, "what does twenty-eight mean?"

Ski, embarrassed, pulled his sleeve down to cover the tattoo. "That was my regiment," he said quietly. "The Twenty-eighth Infantry. I was a corpsman."

"Where were you stationed?" I asked.

He shrugged. "Here and there," he said. "In Nam, mostly."

In Nam. The war had long since ended; but even then, if you wanted to open some wounds, start talking about Viet Nam. Ski knew that. That's probably why he never mentioned it.

I had been ambivalent about the war in Viet Nam. Like most middle-class white kids I supported it at first. The U.S. was doing what it was supposed to do: stopping the spread of evil. My dad's generation had to stop Hitler, mine had to stop Ho Chi Minh; otherwise, LBJ told us, the communists would conquer all of Asia—and then set their sights on us.

But there remained the question of precisely *who* was going to stop this communist juggernaut. It wasn't middle-class white kids. We were given student deferments. We went to college and drank beer while the kids from the vocational high schools and the ghetto high schools were hauled off to some godforsaken jungle on the other side of the world.

Meanwhile guys like me stood on the sidelines with a beer in one hand and a red, white, and blue pom-pom in the other giving the old college cheer: "Go GIs! Beat Commies!" If a few soldiers had to die, well, that was the price of freedom. Implicit, of course, was the understanding that this price would be paid by others, not by us.

I wondered if I could get Ski to talk about those days.

"So what was it like, Ski?" I asked as I dipped the first plaster roll in the bucket. "Being in Viet Nam, I mean."

Ski looked at me before he answered. "It was a hellhole, Doc," he began. "It was hot and dirty and oppressive and full of people who didn't want to be there. Everyone had a chip on his shoulder. I was lucky, though, I was a corpsman. I actually liked that part.

"I lived through a pretty shitty time in Nam. Corpsmen are sent where the action is, so I saw a lot of guys burned up and blown apart and shot to shit. Every day I was surrounded by it."

I finished applying the first roll of plaster, then began working on the second one.

"Yeah," Ski said quietly, "it was a shitty time. I saw so many terrible things over there. I spent every day bandaging and splinting and cauterizing. It became mechanical after a while. I could do it without thinking about it. I didn't *want* to think about it. I just wanted to get it done, serve out my hitch, and go home."

"Yes," I murmured, "I know what you mean."

"But I was wrong, Doc," he said as he expertly shifted his hands away from the plaster as I rolled it. "I had forgotten about those poor grunts who were getting shot to shit for no reason. It's bad enough to get shot or killed for noble purposes, but we didn't know what the hell we were fighting for. Everyone in Nam hated us and everyone at home was embarrassed by us or ashamed of us.

"Nam started to get to me. I drank a lot and smoked a lot of dope, and I probably would have wound up in the guardhouse or rehab if I hadn't finally realized that what those guys needed from me was not just bandaging and splinting and cauterizing. They needed to know that someone cared—not just cared about their leg or their burn or their fitness to return to duty, but cared *about them*. It wasn't just about bandaging wounds—any more than what we did here tonight was about realigning bones." He slipped those last few words in casually, but I knew they were meant for me.

"Right," I said, nodding affirmatively. But while pretending to agree with him, I wondered what he was talking about. What does he mean it isn't about realigning bones?

While my hands were running over the surface of the cast, smoothing the finish, my mind was twisting and turning away from the truth Ski had thrust in front of me. Of course it's about realigning bones. Isn't that what the father brought the kid here for? Isn't that my job?

I am a dumb shit, I realized finally. Of course that isn't my job. I have been missing the boat.

Ski had identified exactly what had been bothering me. I had been failing to see the big picture. I had been developing into an adept technician, learning to repair tendons and reduce bones, but I had forgotten what brought me to medicine in the first place. It wasn't reducing fractures and replacing hips. Those were the means, and I had let them become the ends.

I was stunned, lost, bewildered. I stood there mindlessly rubbing my hands up and down the now-hard cast. Ski covered for me. He motioned to the tech to shoot the post-reduction films. He must have wondered what happened to Captain Efficiency who stood there rubbing a dry cast instead of rushing the tech to get the films done. I stepped back and stood there dumbly, while Ski positioned the arm for the X-ray.

I had let my work become automatic, forgetting the essence of what a doctor is called to do. I had let pragmatism take me too far, take me to where I had lost sight of my calling. I was wrapped up in the technical aspects of what I was doing while ignoring the fact that my vocation wasn't approximating collagen bundles or correcting angulations, it was helping people—living, breathing, hurting people. How could I have forgotten that? Why, even the X-ray tech knew it intuitively, knew enough to show an injured little kid that someone cared about him—and all I could think of was hurrying him up, straightening his arm, and getting on to the next order of business.

The films were back in five minutes. Ski snapped them up on the view box. "Very nice reduction, Doc—as usual." Why had I never noticed the irony in his voice before?

"You can wake him up, Bonnie," I said quietly to the anesthesiologist.

When the boy started to awaken, we wheeled him to the recovery room. While I waited for him to come to, I took Goofy and wrapped a small bit of plaster around his arm, then fashioned a little sling out of Kerlex and tied it around his neck.

"Don't be afraid, Danny," I said as his eyelids fluttered open and he looked about in panic. "We're all done. Your arm is all fixed. And look, we fixed Goofy, too."

He reached with his good arm and I handed Goofy to him.

"Would you like me to get your mom and dad?" I asked him.

"I want my mommy," he answered, his lip quivering.

"You're all fixed, kiddo," I repeated. "We're going to let you and Goofy go home in just a little while."

I picked up the chart and looked at his name: *Oestmann, Daniel. 1451 Cottonwood Avenue, Byron, Minnesota.* I wiped the dried plaster from my forearm, picked up the X-rays, and went out to talk to the parents.

"Hi, Mr. and Mrs. Oestmann," I said. "Danny is fine. Everything went well. His fracture is back in place. He should be able to go home with you tonight."

"Did you have to open it?" his father asked.

"No, sir. I was able to push it back into place without opening it."

His parents beamed. When had I stopped noticing things like that? When had I become so impatient to impart my news, deliver my instructions, and be off?

"Please," I said, gesturing at the couch behind them, "sit down."

I sat with the Oestmanns for fifteen minutes. They told me they had two other children, ten and twelve.

"So Danny's your baby, huh?" I asked Mrs. Oestmann.

"You got that right, Doc," Mr. Oestmann interrupted. "Nancy thinks the earth revolves around him."

"Oh, I do not," Mrs. Oestmann said with a shy smile.

I told them what to watch for, gave them instructions about getting a follow-up X-ray with us in the clinic next week, and asked them to call if they had any concerns. Then I said I was going to see if the recovery-room nurses would let them come back and be with Danny.

They got to their feet and shook my hand. "Thanks, Doc," Mr. Oestmann said. "Thank you so much." I said good night to them and headed back to the recovery room.

I was about to enter my final year of training, but I had learned a valuable lesson that night. When I finished talking to the nurses I headed back to the cast room. There was someone there I needed to thank.

# YEAR FOUR

# CHAPTER THIRTY-THREE

*July*

I was thirty-three years old. I had twenty-seven years of education behind me. I had friends, guys my own age, who were halfway to their pension—and I was still in training. But the end was in sight. On July 2 I began my final year. I was back on Antonio Romero's service, this time as the senior resident. This was it, the last lap.

But Barlow's grocery store, and Jensen's Standard station, and Northwest Bank didn't care how many laps I had left, or how many years of education I had behind me. They wanted to be paid. And for the thirty-third year in a row, I was broke, still living paycheck to paycheck. If it hadn't been for moonlighting we never would have made it.

I was nearing the end of a thirty-six-hour moonlighting stint at St. Joe's: 7:00 P.M. Friday 'til 7:00 A.M. Sunday. Although I had managed a couple hours' sleep each night, I was running on empty. I finished the admission orders, scribbled a signature, then leaned back and ran both hands slowly through my hair.

My last patient had been a seventy-two-year-old lady who had pricked her hand on a rosebush ten days earlier. Although her hand had been infected for a week, she waited until three o'clock in the morning to get it checked. I opened the wound, drained the pus, and discovered a portion of the thorn still inside her.

"Why that little devil," she said when I showed her the thorn.

By the time I finished dressing her hand, starting her on IV antibiotics, and shipping her upstairs, it was time to go home.

I trudged back to the call room and took a quick shower. Jim Leone, who was taking over for me, was already in my bed when I came out of the bathroom.

"Jim," I said, toweling myself dry, "glad to see you're hard at work."

"Leamme alone." He rolled over, pulled up the covers, and faced the wall.

I finished dressing, turned off the light, and said, "Later, Jim. Hope it's quiet."

"See you, Mike," came the muffled reply as the door closed.

As I passed the desk one of the nurses asked me if Dr. Leone was in the call room.

"Yeah. What've you got?"

"An old guy with a painful, red toe."

"Get a CBC, sed rate, uric acid level, and an X-ray and don't wake Dr. Leone 'til they're back."

She nodded and picked up the phone.

As I turned to leave I fell in with the night nurses. They were going off shift, too. We walked to the parking lot together.

"Don't they teach you guys how to shave at Mayo?" Connie Fritz asked, nodding at my unshaven chin. "You look like a bum."

"I'll shave on the way home."

"You'll still look like a bum. Why don't you take a nap before you go?"

"Can't. Gotta meet my wife and kids at Mass at nine."

The nurses laughed. Like everyone else, they thought it was hilarious how we kept having kids. "How many kids do you have now?" Connie asked.

"Three."

"And how old is the oldest?"

"Three."

"God," she said, shaking her head, "your poor wife."

My poor wife. I heard stuff like that every day. I had been up most of the last two nights, had been working roughly forty-nine straight hours, and all I ever heard were things like "your poor wife."

Ah, well, I thought, they're right. Patti does have a pretty hard life—and she deserves better.

Me? Hell, I was just a mule. I was born to work. I slept when I could, then got up and worked some more. And it honestly didn't bother me. I was too pragmatic to let it bother me. Whether it bothered me or not I had to do it. It was better to concentrate on the task at hand.

It was a warm July morning so I didn't have to worry about the car starting. I tossed my books and shaving kit in the backseat. It felt so good to sit down. Maybe a nap wasn't such a bad idea. Just for a few minutes, that's all. I yawned and closed my eyes.

As my head nodded forward, I snapped open my eyes. *Bullshit!* If I fell asleep I wouldn't wake up until noon. I took a deep breath, and started the car. The old Battleship rumbled into life and I swung her out of the parking lot.

I sped down the silent Sunday morning streets, flying in and out of the dark shadows of the old elm trees. When I got to Highway 14 I turned right—directly into the rising sun.

Oh, great, I thought. I'm having a hard time keeping my eyes open as it is.

The sun was too low for the visor to do any good. I crept eastward through the city until I reached the last stoplight in Mankato. When the light turned green I opened up the Battleship and headed into open country, cruising along at about seventy. As I neared Janesville I blew past a mile-long string of railroad cars stopped next to the tall Harvest States grain elevator.

I continued to squint as I headed into the rising sun, and I couldn't stop yawning. With each yawn, my eyes filled with tears. This wasn't good. I had to do something. I rolled down my window and turned up the radio full blast.

*"Breakin' rocks in the hot sun,"* I sang at the top of my voice. *"I fought the law and the law won."* I kept my left hand out the window, slapping a beat on the side of the car as I sped past undulating fields of corn.

A few miles from Waseca my head nodded and the car swerved onto the shoulder. The bumping of the tires on the gravel snapped me awake and frightened the hell out of me. Jesus Christ, I thought, I'm going to kill myself.

I stopped the car, got out, and ran in place for half a minute trying to get the blood flowing again. I flapped my arms across my chest and did some deep knee bends.

My brothers had recently warned me that if I got myself killed "driving around in that shit bucket of yours" they weren't going to raise my kids for me.

"We'll sell 'em to the Gypsies, take the money, and go to Vegas," Tim told me.

"Yeah, we could probably get three, four hundred bucks apiece for them," Denny added.

"Maybe more for the little fat one," Jack said, rubbing his chin and staring appraisingly at Patrick.

I rolled down every window in the car this time, then took off my shirt and drove bare-chested. I decided to leave my pants on, though. I didn't want to risk getting arrested by the Rochester police when I got to church: "PERVERT ARRESTED ON WAY TO MOLEST LADIES OF ALTAR AND ROSARY SOCIETY—Naked doctor arraigned on charges of indecent exposure." How would I explain *that* to BJ Burke?

I pulled the Battleship back onto the road, my head bouncing to the throbbing music. *"Gloria! G-L-O-R-I-A. Glo-ri-a!"*


I was supposed to meet Patti at church at nine. She was going to get a ride from Mrs. Flaherty whose daughter, Mary, often sat for us. It was ten after nine when I swung into the St. Pius parking lot. Unfortunately, an elderly couple arrived at the same time and parked right next to me.

"George, that man is—"

"This way, Margaret, quickly," the man said, hustling his wife away from the demented, bare-chested drug fiend as quickly as he could.

I put on my shirt, ran a hand through my hair, and walked into church. Patti, as always, was sitting in the back row. The girls were sitting next to her. Patrick was squirming on her lap. I whispered hello to them all and squeezed in the pew with them.

During Mass I could hardly keep my eyes open. At the Kiss of Peace, Patti said she hoped I didn't get whiplash from the way my head kept dropping down on my chest.

When Mass was over we gathered up the kids, the toys, the sandwich bag of crushed Cheerios, and the parish bulletin. I had Patrick in my arms and a diaper bag slung over my shoulder. Patti had each of the girls by the hand.

"Why is that couple looking at you like that?" Patti asked.

George and Margaret, grasping each other's arms, were plastered against the wall of the church staring at me with wide eyes.

They seemed like nice people. I knew I should apologize to them, but what would I say? How could I make them understand why a thirty-three-year-old man would show up for church with no shirt on? "Well you see I'm a resident at Mayo and I want to be a good doctor but we have all these kids and we have no money so I have to moonlight and I don't get much sleep but I still want to go to Mass with my family because I want to be a good father even though I'm hardly ever home so I drive ninety miles into the sun but I can't keep my eyes open because I haven't been to bed for two days and my car almost goes off the road so I take off my shirt and turn up the radio and . . ." I stopped. How could I explain my life to them when I didn't even understand it myself?

"Come on, sweetheart," Patti said, tugging my arm. "You look beat, you poor thing. Let me get you home to bed."

To bed. Yes. That much I did understand. I needed to go to bed. I handed Patti the keys and followed her to the car.

# CHAPTER THIRTY-FOUR

*September*

The whole thing started with an innocent remark by Frank Wales.

"You know," he said, studying the flock of geese that had just landed at the other end of the lake, "if a man had a mind to, he could get himself one of those big old birds."

It had been an unseasonably warm September—a long, lingering month with warm fields of corn glowing in the sun against a backdrop of yellow, orange, and red trees. Frank and I were lying crosswise in a rubber raft on the old flooded quarry a mile west of Rochester. Frank's legs were over the right side, mine over the left. A cooler with the remains of a twelve-pack was between us. Our fishing rods, half-forgotten, dangled over either side.

I was a city boy, born and raised on the West Side of Chicago. I knew nothing about farming or fishing or hunting. I had never driven a tractor or owned a gun. But Frank, and many of my fellow residents, had been fishing and hunting for as long as they could remember.

It was Frank's idea to go fishing. It was my idea to bring the beer. I thought I was being innovative, only to learn later that alcohol is an indispensable part of the fisherman's armamentarium.

"If you ain't drunk, you ain't fishin'" is the Minnesota fisherman's creed.

Frank and I had parked my car behind a large bush, hoping to make it less noticeable from the road. The quarry had the usual allotment of signs, all of which were peppered with bullet and shotgun holes: no parking, no fishing, no swimming, no hunting, no trespassing, no dumping, no boating.

We took turns pumping up the raft, then hoisted the cooler and fishing gear aboard and shoved off. It was a warm evening, the sun just setting. Frank brought his surefire bait: a can of Green Giant Niblet Corn. He fastened a piece to his hook, threw it into the water, and almost immediately felt a tug on his line. He reeled in a six-inch, angry-as-hell sunfish that flapped around in the bottom of our raft until Frank tossed him back. No sooner had I dropped my hook in the water than I caught one, this one pushing eight inches.

Within ten minutes we had caught and released fifteen fish. At first we couldn't believe what great fishermen we were, but after the fifteenth fish had committed suicide by impaling itself on our hooks, Frank said, "I've never seen such stupid fish. They'll bite anything"—an opinion that was borne out a few minutes later when we jumped in to swim and felt little fish mouths gumming our toes. After that we just tossed our lines and unbaited hooks into the water, leaned back, drank beer, and watched the stars come out.

"You ever gone goose hunting, Mike?" Frank asked.

"No, I grew up in Chicago, remember? People are more civilized there. They don't shoot animals—only other people. Anyway, isn't there a law against shooting geese around here?"

"Well, yeah," Frank said. "They're protected within a six-mile radius of town. But still, I'd love to shoot one of those fat things. It sure would taste good." He reached into the cooler and took out another beer. "And I know how you could do it without getting caught."

"How?"

"With a twenty-two."

"A *twenty-two*?" I didn't know much about hunting, but I knew you hunted birds with shotguns, not rifles.

"Yeah," Frank said, "a twenty-two. A shotgun is too loud, attracts too much attention. You snuggle up in the weeds with a twenty-two, wait 'til those suckers land, 'til they're sitting real still, and then"—he sighted along his index finger—"pow! Fresh goose for dinner."

Two weeks later, an hour before sunset, I was limping down the side of the road, heading toward the quarry. I had Frank's .22 shoved down my right pant leg.

"Are you out of your mind?" Patti had said when I was leaving. "Poaching is against the law."

"Relax. I'm not going to get caught."

"That's what every crook thinks until he gets arrested."

"Well, this is not a good law. Ask the farmers. They're always complaining about geese destroying their crops."

"So how many farmers do you think are going to get out of bed to bail you out of jail at three o'clock in the morning?"

"I told you, I'm not going to get caught."

"Yes, you are, because I'm going to turn you in. I'll get a hundred bucks for it. Ever heard of T-I-P?" Patti was referring to the *Turn In Poachers* ad on TV sponsored by the Minnesota Department of Conservation.

"Come on, hon. Frank says it'll be a piece of cake. I'll plug the thing and be home in a couple hours. Have you ever tasted fresh goose?"

"Have you ever tasted SOS in the county jail? Because that's where you're going."

I found a spot in the thickest part of the weeds along the western shore of the quarry, hunkered down, and waited. Just as the sun was setting a flock of twelve geese circled once, banked, and landed with a soft splash on the opposite side of the lake. They fluffed their feathers, settled down, and began slowly drifting toward me.

I waited until they were almost to my side of the lake. I carefully pushed aside a couple weeds, lifted my rifle, took aim at the closest goose, and fired. There was a sudden furious honking and flapping of wings as the panicked flock took flight. They rose into the dusk, and in twenty seconds were scarcely visible a quarter mile away. I stood up, my rifle dangling in the crook of my left arm. With my right hand I brushed the damp dirt and twigs from the front of my jacket. It was growing dark now, but on the smooth surface of the silent lake, forty feet offshore, I could see the white breast of the goose I had just killed.

It was the first time I had ever shot another living creature. I felt no elation, no triumph, just a feeling that I had done something wrong, a feeling very close to shame. I had killed something.

I tried to reason with myself. *Do you feel shame every time you eat a hamburger?*

No, I didn't.

*So other people can kill animals for you to eat, but you can't?*

It just didn't seem right to kill an animal like that—when I really didn't have to. It wasn't fun. It wasn't exciting. It was just . . . wrong.

It was darker now, and growing cold. The goose was forty feet offshore, and it was too cold to swim for it. I would have to go home and get the raft.

Thirty minutes later I had pumped up the raft and rowed out to retrieve my goose. I grabbed it by the neck and dropped it into the raft. I was surprised how heavy it was.

When I got back home I walked in the back door, goose in hand, and called Patti.

"Woman of the house, your big hunk o' man is home with food for the family."

Patti came into the kitchen, took one look at me, and immediately held up her hand. "Oh, no you don't. Get that filthy thing out of here."

I was shocked. Is this how the alpha male, the provider, is welcomed back to the cave? "Pat, it's a fresh goose. It's meat."

"It is *not* meat! Meat is something you buy in a grocery store, and it comes wrapped in cellophane. *That*," she said, pointing at my goose, "is a dead animal. Now get that thing out of here before the kids see it. They won't sleep for a month."

"What about the dead skunk and raccoon I have in the trunk?"

She folded her arms and glared at me. "I left my mother and father and a perfectly good home—*for this?* Some nutcase who thinks he's Conan the Barbarian and brings roadkill into my kitchen?"

"Let me clean and pluck this goose and then let's see what you say."

I went out to the garage and laid the goose on the floor, then went back to the basement and got my Buck knife and my dissection kit from first-year Anatomy.

I had never cleaned and dressed an animal before, but I was a doctor, so I had a rough idea what needed to be done. First, I thought, I'll have to pluck it. How hard can that be?

An hour later, a half-bald goose rested on a newspaper in the center of the garage. Feathers were strewn everywhere. I pulled out a pair of latex gloves from my suture laceration kit. Now I would have to clean the damn thing.

Well, I thought, I'll do a midline laparotomy incision followed by a total gastrectomy, duodenectomy, ileectomy, jejunectomy, and colectomy. And if there is anything else left in the abdominal cavity I'll take that out, too. Oh, yeah, the neck and legs, they'll have to go, too.

After another hour I had filled a plastic garbage bag with enough offal to keep every raccoon in Rochester happy for a week. It was ten o'clock. Patti should still be awake. I carried my prize up the back steps only to find the latch was on the door. An oversight on Patti's part, no doubt. I knocked gently on the door.

"Pat," I called. "Patti."

A voice from the hallway answered. "If you have that thing with you, you're not getting in."

"Patti, come on, let me in. It's cleaned and plucked and ready for cooking. Just come and look at it."

She came around the corner in her bathrobe, undid the latch, and quickly stepped back. I opened the door, and held out the goose. She took one look at the gory mess resting on the soggy newspaper in my hands and gagged.

"Oh, God, how could you?"

She looked like she was going to be sick. I started to put the goose on the table and go to her.

"Don't you dare!" she shouted. "Don't you put that thing on my table. Get it out. Right now! I mean it, Michael. Get it out of here or I'll throw up on you."

The left side of her body was trying to go back to the hallway while the right side was trying to push me out the back door. Under ordinary circumstances it would have been an amusing spectacle to watch. However, having been married for five years, and being a quick learner, I realized the combination of revulsion, disgust, hatred, and anger on her face meant Patti was not pleased. The revulsion and disgust would disappear if I took my goose and left the room. The hatred and anger I would have to deal with later.

I backed out the door and trudged wearily back to the garage.

Now what? Where was I going to put the goose? Patti wouldn't let me keep it in the house. But if I left it in the garage, squirrels and raccoons would eat it. That left . . . the backseat of the car! Yeah, that's it. Just for the night. I'd get it out first thing in the morning before Patti woke up.

I set the carcass on the hood and then opened the back door of the car. One of the kid's car seats was belted down. I couldn't find the buckle in the dark so I went back to the hood, got the goose, and set it in the car seat. I made sure all the windows were closed, slammed the door, and went to bed.


At six o'clock the next morning, Saturday, Eileen came into our bedroom and pressed her face into Patti's.

"Mom?"

Patti opened her left eye ten percent. "Huh?"

"Something happened to Mary Kate."

The eye opened another ten percent. "*What* happened to Mary Kate?"

"She got shrunked."

Patti shifted a little under the covers and let out a sigh. "What do you mean, 'she got shrunked'?"

"She's in her car seat and she got shrunked. And she doesn't smell so good."

Oh, Jesus, I thought as I sprang out of bed. I'm screwed now. "Never mind, Eileen," I said as I yanked on a pair of sweatpants. "Daddy will take care of it."

Patti slowly sat up and turned on me. I didn't like the look in her eyes. It was the same look Godzilla gave Tokyo before he fire-breathed it.

"You didn't," she said.

I couldn't look at her. "Relax, hon, it's probably nothing. You know how kids are. Heh-heh. I'll just run out and see what Eileen's talking about."

I was out the door before I could hear everything she was saying, but the words "Michael" and "kill you" were repeated several times in gradually increasing volume. I tore out to the garage, whipped the goose out of Mary Kate's car seat, stuck it in the wheelbarrow, and covered it with a bag of fertilizer. Unfortunately there was a spot of goose juice on the car seat and an unmistakable smell of the great outdoors.

I turned and walked back to the house. Patti was waiting at the back door.

"Well?" she said.

There are times to lie, to shamelessly and obstinately lie, to deny everything, to look your wife right in the eye and swear black is white.

This was not one of those times.

All I could do was to throw myself on the mercy of the court. Court was in session, but the Honorable Attila the Hun was presiding. Patti was shocked, horrified, outraged. How could I have done such a thing? What could I possibly have been thinking? Poor Eileen would be scarred for life because of this.

"I don't know where that filthy thing is," she said, presumably referring to the goose, not Eileen, "but I never want to see it again."

I was told if I cared anything, anything at all, about my wife and children I would get rid of that disgusting thing this minute. "And don't come back until you do!" Then the back door slammed.

I got the picture.

I wrapped the goose in a plastic garbage bag and brought it to Jack Manning who was going up to St. Paul to see his sister. He promised to drop it off at my brother Pete's apartment.

Pete called a few days later to say he and his roommates stuffed and cooked the goose. "It was the best meal we've had all year," he said. "It was really nice of you and Patti to send it to us."

"No problem."

"Be sure to thank Patti for us, too."

That is one message that has never been delivered.

# CHAPTER THIRTY-FIVE

*November*

When we finished our last case I let Charlie Norrie go. He had been up all night and was dead on his feet. "Go home, Charlie," I told him. "I'll take care of rounds." He was too tired to argue. He lifted a hand in thanks and was gone.

I was the senior resident on Tom Hale's service. Charlie was the junior resident. Tom was one of the young guns of the Mayo program. He was smart. He had great hands, and he let his residents do a lot of operating. Every resident at Mayo wanted to be on his service. Charlie and I were thrilled to get the chance to spend a quarter with him.

We had twenty-one patients on our service, most of them recovering from major surgery: joint replacements, fractures, osteotomies, cuff repairs. We had patients in casts, braces, and traction; patients bleeding, draining, and vomiting; patients with high fevers, low blood counts, and weak pulses. It was challenging, daunting almost, but I approached each patient methodically, putting everything else out of my mind, trying to figure out exactly what was wrong and exactly what needed to be done.

I had been insecure for so long, that even now, despite all I had learned, I still suspected I wasn't as good as the other residents; consequently I forced myself to be so thorough that nothing would get by me.

My insecurity had served me well. It incited me, it drove me, and it kept me persevering when fatigue or common sense would have made me stop. But it was also changing me in some not-so-pleasant ways. I was becoming almost obsessive about studying every night. I *had* to know everything about every problem in every patient.

As usual it was Patti who helped me keep things in perspective. She knew when to encourage me to work, and she knew when to send one of the kids down to my office in the basement to "tell Daddy to put his books away. We're going to the park now."

It took me three hours to make rounds without Charlie. When I finally finished, I dropped the last few charts on the desk at the nursing station. As I sat down, I noticed a framed picture on the wall behind the med cart. It was the photograph of a young woman, taken from behind. She was standing next to a tree, on the crest of a hill, with a vast landscape opening in front of her. Her hair was blowing in the breeze. It was a striking picture. I looked at it for a second or two before I realized the woman was on crutches. She had only one leg.

"Do you like the picture, Doctor?" one of the nurses asked.

"Yeah. It's nice." Nice, but disconcerting. A beautiful girl—but she was missing a leg.

"That's Sarah Berenson. She was one of our patients."

Sarah Berenson. Perhaps I gasped, I'm not sure.

The nurse must have seen my distress. "Do you know her?"

Sarah Berenson. Oh, God, how I despised myself at that moment. Did I know her? I helped Bill Kramer take off her leg. For months after her surgery I had been unable to get the vision of Sarah out of my mind. Sarah, her blond hair tousled on her pillow, her breasts nudging against the flowered hospital gown. Sarah, with that childlike light in her eyes, the light no amount of suffering had ever been able to dampen. Sarah was the girl I had sworn I would never forget.

Another broken promise. I *had* forgotten.

I realized that it had been close to a year since I had even thought of

Sarah. How, I wondered, could I so completely forget someone who meant so much to me, whom I had sworn I would *never* forget?

Sometimes I am not the most perceptive of men, and I had actually made a mental note to reread the section on memory in my old neurology text. But at that point something clicked in me, and I realized that there was no way I could have let Sarah slip through the cracks of my memory. I must have crammed her through the cracks myself. I must have pushed and squeezed and jammed her out of my memory. I must have realized that, in my profession, there were going to be a lot of Sarahs, and if I kept erecting shrines to them in my memory, if I kept lighting candles in front of those shrines, the conflagration eventually would burn me up.

I must have wondered about Sarah. I certainly cared about how she was doing. And yet I never made an effort to follow up on her. I never asked Bill Kramer about her. I knew Annie Cheevers, the nurse who cared for her post-op, kept in touch with her, but I never asked Annie, either.

Why? I wondered. It wasn't that I didn't care. I cared a lot about Sarah. Maybe that was it, maybe I cared too much. Maybe I was afraid of what I might find out if I asked too many questions. Maybe I suspected what the answer might be.

Well, I wasn't going to hide from it anymore. I would call Annie Cheevers that night and ask her how Sarah was.


But it turned out I didn't need to call Annie, for at that moment, the nurse standing next to me said, "Sarah died a few months ago. She was the sweetest girl. We all loved her."

I suppose I knew it all along. I suppose that was what I had been hiding from this past year. I looked at the picture, watching the way Sarah's hair drifted in the breeze. I wondered what she had been thinking as she looked out on that vast panorama of life that opened before her. She knew, of course, for her it wasn't opening at all.

*She died a few months ago.*

That meant Sarah lived for about a year after her surgery. So what the hell had we done for her? We took off her leg. We put her through a terrible amount of pain. And for what? She died anyway. Did our surgery do anything for her? Did it lengthen her life, or shorten it? I wondered if she would have been better off if she had never heard of the Mayo Clinic. We did the best we could, but for the hundredth time I realized that doing the best we could wasn't enough. There was something in me that wanted results not just effort. Don't tell me how hard you tried, tell me whether or not you succeeded.

I couldn't hold back. I began to bludgeon myself. Let me get this straight, I sneered at myself. A beautiful, young girl came to you. You cut off her leg, ripped out her pelvis, and spilled most of the blood in her body. Then you gave her poison that made her hair fall out, made her blood cells die, and made her vomit until her esophagus bled. Then you radiated her until you killed every egg in her ovaries. And you kept all that up until she was dead. But you insist it was the *cancer* that killed her. And despite all that happened, despite all you did, everything is supposed to be okay because "you meant well." Huh. Do me a favor, Doctor, if I ever get sick stay the hell away from me with your good intentions.


Thank God for the successes. Thank God for the people whose hips and knees we replaced, who showered us with gratitude. Thank God I didn't have to go home every night wondering if anything I did mattered a goddamn. I couldn't do it. I couldn't handle a steady stream of failure and death.

Maybe that's why I "forgot" Sarah. Maybe it was just too much for me.

# CHAPTER THIRTY-SIX

*January*

We spent Christmas in Chicago, then drove back to Rochester on New Year's Day in a blizzard. It was midnight before we finally arrived home. The car got stuck halfway up the driveway so I just left it there.

I was up early the next morning, anxious to get going. It was a special day. I was going to begin my final assignment at the Mayo Clinic: chief resident in Orthopedic Surgery. I would have my own service with my own patients. I would do all my own cases, and would have a junior resident assigned to me.

I should have been proud and thrilled. This was the culmination of everything I had worked for since I was a junior resident on Dr. Harding's service three and a half years earlier. Unfortunately I took very little pleasure in being selected chief resident. I was no longer programmed for pleasure. I was programmed for achievement. Rather than spending a little time basking in the glory, I immediately moved on to planning my next achievement: becoming a good, no an *excellent,* chief resident. I began calculating what I should do and how I should do it.

I told Patti I was worried. Being chief resident was a big responsibility and I didn't want to screw up. She brushed away my concerns. "You're awesome," she said. "You'll do great." Of course, if I wanted to be Emperor of Japan Patti would tell me I was awesome and I'd do great.

As I finished shaving I looked at Patti's bathrobe, floppy slippers, and disheveled hair. "Lookin' good," I said.

She pushed the hair back from her face. "Feelin' good," she replied with a smile.

She bent over, picked up a rubber dinosaur, and stuffed it in the pocket of her bathrobe. As she wrapped the robe around her, I noticed it was getting a little tight—again. She was due with our fourth child in May.

"You can kiss that Planned Parenthood Man of the Year award goodbye now," Bill Chapin had said when he heard the news.

"Unregulated animalistic breeding," Patti's liberated, older sister had said when she heard the news.

"Who cawes?" our son Patrick had said when he heard the news.

As I put on my L.L. Bean parka and Sorrel boots, I noticed the streets had been plowed, but a wall of snow now blocked my exit from the driveway. I wasn't worried, though. I knew the old Battleship would get me through.

I called good-bye to the kids who were down in the basement destroying things. They came thundering up the stairs. Eileen said Mary Kate took her crayons. Mary Kate said Patrick hit her with a hockey stick. Patrick said Mary Kate was "a alien," and he was going to "vapowize her." Patti grabbed the hockey stick and said she would vaporize them all if they didn't knock it off.

"Have a nice day, dear," I said over the din as I zipped my coat and started out the door.

She stuck out her tongue at me. "Close the door, you big omadhaun," she said. "We're all going to get pneumonia. It's freezing out."

"Yeah," Patrick said, "it's fweezing out."

"You big omadhaun!" Eileen giggled as I shut the door.

I crunched through the snow to the car, listening to everyone inside laughing. ("You called Dad an omadhaun!") They were gathered in the living-room window, climbing all over each other, waving and pointing as I revved up the Battleship and sent it flying down the driveway, smashing through the wall of snow, and skidding into the snowbank on the opposite side of the street. I waved to the kids, gunned the engine, and fishtailed down the street.

Alan Harkins, the senior resident assigned to me, was waiting when I got to the doctors' lounge at St. Mary's. Alan was a quiet, studious guy who didn't play hockey, didn't play golf, drank wine instead of beer, and preferred The Amsterdam Concertgebouw to the Clancy Brothers. On the surface we didn't have a lot in common. We did, however, share one important trait: we were both very serious about our work.

When we finished rounds I told Alan he could have Sunday off. I would make rounds by myself. He, of course, demurred, but I insisted.

"I'll see you at seven Monday morning," I said. "And I'll be around all weekend, so call me if you have any problems."

When Alan had gone I went to the residents' lounge to check the bulletin board for practice opportunities. In six months my residency would be over. I needed to find a job. One good thing about being a resident at Mayo is that there is never a shortage of job offers: Seattle, Colorado, Chicago, Tampa, Dallas, Boston. I pretty much had my pick of places. It felt strange to be looking for a job. Even though I was now chief resident, I still felt as if I had just started, and now I was making plans to leave.

Although I was eager to begin my work as chief resident, there was one thing that bothered me. It is traditional that the chief resident let his resident do a lot of surgery. Only jerks hog all their cases. I knew Alan expected me to turn over a lot of my cases to him, but this was going to be hard for me. Hell, I had just started getting comfortable doing cases myself, and now I had to let a less-experienced resident do them—in my name? If Alan screwed up, it was *my* reputation that was on the line. It was *my* patient who would be harmed. I didn't know if I was ready for that.

The issue of residents doing cases had come to a head in our department the year before when Bill Chapin was on Don Ashford's service. Ashford was new on staff and was still insecure about letting residents do cases. His residents rarely got to do any surgery. Bill didn't like it, and never one to back down from anything, he took his complaints to BJ Burke, insisting that something be done.

"Either this is a training program, or it's not," Bill insisted. "And if it is, then residents have to operate."

Ashford took the moral high ground, insisting that "patient care" came first, and that "our mission to provide proper patient care takes precedence over our mission to train residents."

Ashford had pressed the right button and he knew it. Everyone at the Clinic paid lip service to the notion that patient care came first, even though everyone knew that wasn't always true. It was one of those uncomfortable truths easier to ignore than to acknowledge.

The patient did not always come first—especially in the surgical specialties. If the Mayo Clinic's primary concern was patient care, then how could they *ever* let a resident do a case? The resident is virtually never a better surgeon than the attending surgeon. Now that I was chief resident I was pretty good at doing most orthopedic operations. But I never for a moment thought I was better than Antonio Romero or Tom Hale or Mark Coventry. So how could the Clinic justify letting me do cases when everyone knew I wasn't as good as those guys? And how could I justify letting Alan do cases when I knew he wasn't as good as I was?

Residents can't become surgeons unless they do surgery—and everyone knows it. But residents aren't as proficient as attending surgeons—and everyone knows that, too. And yet at every training center in the United States residents do cases; and at every training center in the United States administrators continue to proclaim, "Patient care comes first."

I was sitting in the front seat of Chris Pfeffer's Olds drinking a Grain Belt. It was 11:45 P.M. Hockey had ended fifteen minutes earlier. Chris was a fourth-year ENT resident who had played college hockey at Harvard. He and I usually had a few beers together in the parking lot before heading home. The engine was running and the car was just starting to warm up. We were talking about residents doing surgery.

"I feel like a hypocrite," I told him. "If I truly believed the system was wrong, I should have refused to do any cases these last four years. I should have insisted my attending do every case. Why didn't I have the courage to admit that the attending was a better surgeon than I, and that the patient's right to care was greater than my right to learn? Where were my scruples then? Hell, I did every case I could."

"Me, too," Chris said. "Still do."

"You know what's funny?" I said. "Now that I'm in my last year, I actually *don't* do every case I can. I've already done so many hip and knee replacements that I don't need to do any more. I let the younger guys do them."

Chris took a long pull on his beer and laughed. "I get it," he said. "As long as you don't feel competent doing a case, you do it; but as soon as you get good at it, you turn it over to your junior resident."

"Yeah, what a system. It guarantees that all cases are done by the least competent person—a kind of medical Peter Principle."

"You think too much," Chris said, yawning and tossing me another beer. "You and I don't make the rules. We're just a couple of fucking Zambonis riding up and down the ice. We go where we're pointed. Someone else is at the controls."

"That doesn't mean it's right."

"Jesus, Mike, get off this 'right' stuff will you? Do you want to leave here after four years never having done a case?"

"Well, no."

"Then shut the hell up. Leave it to BJ and the other big shots to figure out all this other shit. How can Chris Pfeffer and Mike Collins sort it all out? Hell, we have enough trouble trying to live on the two-fifty an hour they pay us."

As I drove home that night I wondered if I was being too hard on myself. I turned cases over to my junior resident and taught him, just as my senior residents had turned cases over to and taught me. That was how we learned. But what continued to gnaw at me was the suspicion we ran a system good for *us* under the guise of being good for the patient.

"A little more anteversion. See how I've got the tibia pointing straight up and down? You want the femoral component to be angled just a bit more *that* way."

I was guiding Alan through his first total hip replacement. He had watched me do several cases, and was familiar with the technique. I had gradually let him do more and more. But this was the first case I let him do it all, "skin to skin."

He was nervous, and wanted my input at every step. That's fine, I thought. I'd rather have someone too cautious than too cocky. When the femoral component was cemented in, Alan reduced the hip and put it through a range of motion. Then we set the leg on the Mayo stand and began to close. I could see the relief in Alan's eyes. The hard stuff was over.

"Great job," I told him.

"Very nice, Doctor," Gladys the scrub nurse said.

"Gee, Alan, you must be good. Gladys never says that to me."

"I do, too."

"You do? Then does that mean you think I'm as good as Dr. Coventry?" Everyone knew she worshiped Dr. Coventry.

"Never!" she said immediately. "None of you are." She slapped a hemostat into my hand.

"Not even Jack Manning?" I asked as I cauterized the bleeder.

"Phhht," she said. "Dr. Manning." She spat out his name, but it was all part of the game we played. She loved Jack, but she hated the way he teased her about how he was going to be the "next" Dr. Coventry.

The post-op X-ray looked great. I had the techs make an extra copy for Alan. Gladys, Nita the circulator, and I all signed it for him.


Alan and I had been working together for a month and things had been going well. I was at home changing the oil in the Battleship when Patti told me Alan was on the phone. We were on call that weekend. That meant Alan would initially handle any injuries or consults. He would call me if he needed help or advice.

"Mike," he said, "I'm in the ER. We've got a sixty-two-year-old lady with a mid-shaft femur fracture, an open Colles, a fracture-dislocation of the ankle, and a shitload of belly and head trauma."

"Car crash?"

"No, attempted suicide. She jumped out a window."

Suicide. We didn't see much of that in Rochester. I asked if she was stable.

"Not really. Her pressure is sixty or so. The general surgeons are taking her to the OR now. They said we can do our part when they're done."

I told Alan I would be right there. I finished filling the Battleship with oil and drove to the ER. Alan introduced me to the family. The specter of suicide lay all over them. They were by turn embarrassed, apprehensive, angry, and hurt. Apparently she was an alcoholic and had brought more than her share of trouble to the family. I found it hard to tell if they were more upset that she attempted suicide or that she failed. They didn't seem terribly interested in what her injuries were or what we were going to do about them.

It was almost 5:00 P.M. before the general surgeons finished exploring the belly. They removed her spleen and repaired her liver. It was ten by the time Alan and I had rodded her femur, plated her ankle, put a lag screw across her talus, and externally fixed her distal radius. We took her to the ICU where she promptly coded. She died an hour later.

I went out to break the news to the family. The waiting room was empty. They had all gone home.

What a waste, I thought. What a total waste.

I had worked so hard to put her back together. I wanted everything to be perfect. I made sure we got the correct rotation and length of the femur. I made sure we got an anatomic reduction of the lateral malleolus. I made sure we avoided devascularizing the talus. I made sure we put the ex-fix on the radius just right. Her post-op films looked great.

Yeah, I thought, she'll have the best-looking X-rays in the morgue.

Sitting there alone in the doctors' locker room, head bowed, hands in my lap, I found it all so pointless. I had used all my skill and training to fix a lady whose family didn't care about her, who didn't care about herself, and who only lived for one hour.

I tried to give myself the usual pep talk: you do the best you can. What happens after that is beyond your control. But pep talks weren't working that night. It was one of those nights when everything seems absurd, when everything seems so laughably presumptuous. What difference would it have made if she had lived another day, another year, another decade? In the end nothing would change.

I'm an orthopod, I thought. I fix things. Big deal. Everything I fix winds up in a coffin anyway.

# CHAPTER THIRTY-SEVEN

*March*

As our fourth Minnesota winter dragged to a close, I was starting to feel comfortable as the chief resident. I loved having my own service. It was almost like being a real doctor. But being chief resident also meant being a little schizophrenic. The younger residents thought of me as an attending surgeon. They constantly came to me for advice, wondering how to treat this or repair that. But the attending surgeons still thought of me as a resident, a convenient place to dump things. As elsewhere in life, that brown stuff kept flowing downhill—and I had to be there to catch it all. Every goofy case, every undesirable consult, was shunted to the chief resident.

I was sitting at breakfast one morning when Charlie Norrie sat down at our table. Charlie had been the junior resident with me on Antonio Romero's service. He was a hardworking guy from Gary, Indiana, and a lifelong White Sox fan.

Charlie didn't want to talk about the Sox today. "Mike," he said, "I have a consult for you."

Frank Wales, who was sitting next to me, clapped his hands. "A consult for the chief resident," he said. "This'll be good."

"Screw off, Wales," Bill Chapin said. "Quit trying to rain on Collins's parade. Charlie's consult is probably from the head of IBM who needs a total hip. Mike'll do the hip and the guy will be so grateful he'll buy Mike a plane ticket around the world. Isn't that right, Charlie?"

Charlie frowned and said, "Well, no . . . not exactly."

"Let's hear it, Charlie," I said.

He cleared his throat and looked at the notes in front of him. "The patient is a well-developed, well-nourished fifty-six-year-old white female librarian who presents with a chief complaint of—"

"Charlie, save the medical bullshit for the fleas. Just tell me what you've got."

"It's a lady with an infected knee."

I groaned.

"For the sixth time."

Chapin and Wales were nudging each other, snickering. Frank slapped me on the back and said, "Ain't this the dad-gumdest, most perfect chief resident's case in the history of the Mayo Clinic?"

I was used to strange consults. I began telling Bill and Frank about a consult I had seen the month before on a man with shoulder pain. The routine at Mayo is for the junior resident on call to see the consult the night it comes in. He presents it to the chief resident who sees it the next day.

It turned out, though, that the gentleman with shoulder pain was a bigshot lawyer from Philadelphia who wanted everything, and wanted it immediately. As soon as he was admitted to the hospital he started complaining. His room sucked. The hospital sucked. The nurses sucked. They brought him his dinner and (surprise!) it sucked, too, so he dumped it on the floor.

Finally the nurses couldn't put up with him for another minute. Annie Cheevers paged me. She said the man had refused to let the junior resident come in the room. "Please," Annie said, "could you see him tonight? I'm afraid he may hurt someone—and if not, someone here may hurt *him*." Annie had done me a lot of favors over the years so I told her I would come right over.

It was about ten o'clock when I got to St. Mary's. His Eminence was sitting on the edge of his bed, fully dressed. He had refused to put on a hospital gown. He was tapping his foot on the floor, looking at his Rolex.

I didn't even get a chance to introduce myself before he said he'd been waiting for three hours and what the hell did I mean keeping him waiting so long?

I apologized and told him consults usually weren't seen until the next day. When I introduced myself as the chief resident, he was outraged. He didn't want "some piece-of-shit resident." He wanted the chairman of the department. There was nothing I would have liked more than to call Big John Harding at home and tell him to come in. Or better yet, BJ Burke. I would have given anything to see what BJ would say to this gentleman.

I began to take a history but the man wouldn't answer my questions. He got up and began pacing around the room. He said his shoulder had been hurting for over a month. He was tired of it. It felt like Son of Sam was sticking giant daggers in his shoulder every minute of every day.

"Do you understand what I am saying, Doctor?" he said.

I was trying to remember who Son of Sam was. I knew he didn't work for Mother Teresa but I couldn't remember if he was a murderer, or someone from Nixon's cabinet, or who the hell he was.

Suddenly the patient strode across the room, slammed his hand down on my left shoulder, and began digging his fingernails into my skin. "Do you feel that, Doctor Whatever-your-name-is? Well, that is what I am living with every minute of every day, and I want it taken care of. Now!"

Pain shot through my shoulder as he continued digging his nails deeper. His jaw jutted out, only three feet from my clenched right fist. In a setting other than a hospital room I might have responded differently. But retaining my professional decorum, I yanked his hand off my shoulder, got to my feet, and stared him down.

"I am going to leave now," I said slowly, "but before I leave I am going to instruct the nurses to treat you with courtesy and respect. I expect you to treat everyone in this hospital in exactly the same manner."

I went out to the nurses' station where Annie Cheevers had a cup of coffee and some chocolate-chip cookies waiting for me. "Annie," I said, "after what I've been through I need a bottle of Valium." Annie thanked me and then told me to be sure I ordered the world's strongest sleeping pill for him.

At this point Frank Wales interrupted my story. "That's it," he said, slamming his palm on the table. "That's more than any man can be expected to take. It's obvious what that feller needed was TPW."

We all looked at him. "What?"

"It's an old Wyoming folk remedy. We used to use it at home on recalcitrant cases."

"What is it?"

"TPW," he said, slowly nodding his head. "Therapeutic Pistol-Whipping. Nothing too drastic. You just lay the barrel of your six-shooter up against the side of that man's head. Not hard enough to kill him. That would be TPE, Therapeutic Pistol Euthanasia. Too much paperwork after that one. TPW is plenty.

"Of course you also could have tried PPW—Prophylactic Pistol-Whipping. You don't wait for the little worm to start whining. You just walk into the room and lay him out with the barrel of your .45. Then see if Mr. Bigshot isn't a little more respectful when he comes to."

"TPW," I said, nodding thoughtfully and rubbing my chin. "Do you think it's covered under most insurance plans? Maybe I could try it this morning."


I thanked Frank for his advice, and went off to see my consult. Jane Satkamp was a pleasant lady in her late forties. She had contracted polio at an early age, and had been left with a withered left leg. She had some sort of antiquated metal brace that looked like it was made of cast iron and rhinoceros leather. The brace continually rubbed the side of her knee, leaving a raw, draining sore. Just looking at the purulent, dripping mess made me queasy. Jane insisted on wearing the brace because she couldn't walk without it. In addition to the infection, Jane had post-polio syndrome that was slowly and inexorably stealing her strength.

"Couldn't you just use a wheelchair for a few weeks to give this thing a chance to heal?" I asked.

"No," she said, "I couldn't. I seem to be getting weaker and weaker. I'm afraid if I ever stop walking I will never walk again."

Jane and I hit it off right away. She was extremely well read, and we always found a little time each day to discuss some book or author we both admired. I made the mistake one day of mentioning Louis L'Amour, and from then on she continually teased me about my degeneration into "escapist, male-fantasy fiction."

Jane was one of the few patients I ever called by her first name. I had always felt that using a patient's first name was too familiar, that it presumed too much on the part of the surgeon. ("*I* am Dr. Smith, but *you* are Alice.") Ms. Satkamp would have none of it, however. "I insist that you call me Jane," she said. "I feel old enough as it is without having someone in his thirties call me Ms. Satkamp."

I did what I could for Jane. I fought with the Mayo Clinic brace shop about fixing her brace. They had never seen anything like it. It was so old they were afraid it would break if they tried to adjust it. They made her a new one but she didn't like it. She said it didn't support her leg the right way. She went back to the old one.

I told Jane I was going to have to take her to the operating room to debride her wound. On the night before her surgery I asked her if she had a husband or child who might want to speak to me.

She gave me a perplexed look; surprised I would ask such a naive question. "I'm not married," she said.

We were both embarrassed, not by what she had said, but by what her words and tone of voice had implied: "I'm not married. I'm a cripple. Who would have me?"

I could have told her she was talking nonsense. I could have chided her for making such a remark. But, sadly, I knew what she meant. We live in a world preoccupied with appearance. Jane had resigned herself to that fact.

Despite her deformity, Jane was a very pretty woman, and was obviously intelligent and personable. Yes, she had a bad leg, but why, I wondered, is that such a big deal? What fool would reject a woman simply because her left leg didn't look like her right one? Jane was worth twenty symmetrically legged women. But men couldn't get past her withered leg.

I considered how poorly served men are by the Darwinian impulse that drives them to grovel before vacuous, self-absorbed beauties, whose attraction lies not in what they are, but in what they represent.

In my short medical career I had treated many people who had been stricken with a severe illness or deformity at a young age. Few of them had ever married. Life, it seemed, had been doubly unfair to them. Not only were they victims of a terrible disease, but they were also deprived of the solace and comfort of love.

At home that night I told Patti how wrong it all seemed. I had been thinking about my childhood, and I cringed with shame when I recalled how I used to mimic the lurching gate of the spastic, and the thick, guttural speech of the retarded. Later, in high school, my thoughtless cruelty "improved" to a careless disregard. I made the crippled disappear. I saw right through them. I could enter a room and not even let their existence register in my consciousness. They just weren't there. Flushed with youth and strength, I had made the subconscious determination that these people, like cocker spaniels and geraniums, inhabited a lower plane of existence, and did not merit my attention.

"Why do those who look different have such a hard time finding love, or even tolerance, from the rest of us?" I asked aloud.

Patti shook her head. She wondered if it was because the crippled force us to confront our own human frailty. "Maybe they make us realize how fragile our hold on life is. Maybe we resent them for reminding us of truths we would prefer to ignore."

I thought of the festering sore on Jane's knee, and that queasy feeling came back again. Why? I had seen scores, hundreds of worse sights in the last four years. What had that gnarled piece of hardware rubbing away on Jane's withered leg been trying to tell me?

Jane and I fought the good fight, but to no avail. I took her to the operating room four times, but her infection wouldn't heal. Every time she put on the brace it rubbed off the newly formed scab, and the wound would become infected all over again. Finally I told Jane that if she didn't stop using the brace she was going to wind up with an amputation.

Reluctantly, she agreed to use a wheelchair temporarily. It took two months but we finally got the sore on her leg to heal. But two months was all it took for Jane to lose what little leg strength she had left.

She never walked again.

Not for the first time in the last four years, I asked myself what went wrong. I did the best I could, but things didn't turn out right.

"But it's not my fault!" I wanted to scream at the world. "I did what I could. Yes, it's a shame Jane can't walk anymore, but what was I supposed to do, ignore her infection and let her die of sepsis?"

The problem, I realized, lay in my conception of what a doctor should be. I wanted to be the guy people came to when life dealt with them unfairly. I wanted to be the guy who confronted the arbitrariness of life and strangled the unfairness out of it.

Jane knew before she ever met me that life was offering her a choice: die of infection or be stuck in a wheelchair for the rest of her life. She already knew that. She came to me holding that knowledge in her outstretched hands, begging me to make it go away, begging me to make things fair.

I tried, Jane. I tried.

# CHAPTER THIRTY-EIGHT

*May*

> **Pay to the order of Patricia Collins**
> **One Mother's Day**
> **with all the benefits normally associated therewith**
> **Signed, MJ Collins MD**

The sun wasn't even up yet. Patti lay propped in bed opening her Mother's Day cards. The IOU card wasn't that funny. I had done the same thing when I left her alone last Mother's Day.

Our financial situation remained precarious. I had five, soon to be six, mouths to feed, and a chief resident's salary just didn't cut it. I *had* to moonlight, but it was harder to arrange coverage at work, and it was harder to leave Patti. She was nine months pregnant and had three other kids to deal with.

"Sweetheart," I said, taking her hand, "I'm really sorry. I hate to leave you." She grunted and heaved herself up to give me a hug.

"What if I go into labor?" she asked. She was already ten days overdue.

"You call me and I'll get right home. Jack said he'd cover for me if I had to leave."

"Why didn't you ask Jack to take the whole day?"

I got up and began to pace around the room. "Aw, hon, you know why. We need the money. How are we going to pay our bills? How are we going to pay for this baby?"

"It's not fair. The baby keeps kicking me in the ribs, my legs are killing me, and the other kids have been awful—"

"And today is Mother's Day," I said, hoping she could see how ashamed I was to leave her.

"Well, whoop-dee-doo. Happy Mother's Day."

"Patti, I don't know what else to do."

"So you take off and I'm stuck bringing the kids to Mass all by myself."

"I'm not going on a picnic, you know."

She rolled away from me and began to cry. "Oh, I know. But why today? Couldn't you have stayed home this one day?"

"I wish I could stay home *every* day, but I can't. You know that."

"Then just go," she said.

"I'm not going like this, with you mad at me."

"I'm not mad at you," she said, her voice muffled in the pillow.

I came around and lay on the bed next to her. "Patti, I'm so sorry," I said, running my hand through her hair. "To leave you, nine months pregnant, on Mother's Day . . ." I was close to tears myself.

We held each other for several minutes. "I'd better go, sweetheart," I said finally.

"I know."

I kissed her and turned to go.

"See you Monday night?" she asked.

"Yeah," I called over my shoulder, "Monday night."


Three nights later Patti finally went into labor. I had been playing hockey and didn't get home until almost midnight. I showered and went into our bedroom where Patti was lying on her side, both hands on her belly. The light on her side of the bed was on.

"I think I'm going to have our baby," she said quietly as I slipped into bed with her.

She was always so calm, so ready.

"Have our baby—like now?"

"Mmm-hmm."

"All right," I said, springing to my feet and pacing around the room. "Hold on. Just take it easy. Everything's going to be fine." I pointed at the telephone. "I'll call Dawn." Dawn was the nursing student who lived next door. She had agreed to stay with the kids when the time came to have the baby.

"I already called her."

"You did? When?"

"A half hour ago. I told her you would be home from hockey around midnight. She was going to watch for your car."

A minute later the doorbell rang. I let Dawn in and then asked Pat what I should pack for her.

"I already packed everything. It's by the back door," she said, struggling to her feet.

I rushed to her side. "Are you having contractions?" I asked.

"Yes, dear. That's how women have babies."

"Well," I said, reaching for her arm, "is there anything I can do?"

"You already did it," she said, managing a smile.

Two hours later Maureen was born. Kenny Billings, our obstetrician, made it just in time. When it was all over, Jack Manning, who was on call that night, stuck his head in the delivery room, said congratulations, and asked, "Is Patti pregnant again yet?"

Patti said if she could get off the table she would kill him with her bare hands.


Four kids under five. They all thought we were nuts. Maybe we were, but we loved it.

Years later, after Patti almost died giving birth to our twelfth child, her obstetrician told us that was it; that was our last child. "You can have twelve kids and two parents," he said, "or thirteen kids and one. Take your pick."

For years afterward, whenever we would see a couple with a little baby, Patti would put her hand on my arm, tears in her eyes, and we would share the same unspoken wish. If only we could have one more—just one more. We would be so grateful. Just to hold one of those sweet little things in our arms, to feel her skin, to smell her baby smell. We knew we had been lucky. We knew we had been blessed. But if we could just have one more . . .

# CHAPTER THIRTY-NINE

*May*

All of a sudden I was homesick. I had been on the phone talking to my brother Tim. He'd been at Aunt Liz's seventieth birthday party and told me how our cousin Eddie had chugged a beer while standing on his head. He was the hit of the party. We had cousins who were pilots, cops, soldiers, politicians, and lawyers, but no one cared about them. Everyone wanted to see Eddie chug a beer upside down—again, and again, and again.

"About the sixth time," Tim told me, "Eddie's standing there, upside down, when Denny pours a glass of ice water down his pant leg. Eddie gasps and sucks half a beer up his nose. The next day he has the worst headache in the history of mankind."

"Worse than yours the day after Sean Walsh's bachelor party?"

"I told you never to mention that day again. Anyway, Eddie goes to the doctor and finds out he's got a sinus infection. Eddie says it's too bad he wasn't drinking flaming shots: they might have cleared his sinuses right out. The doctor is some Czechoslovakian or Nicaraguan or something. He isn't used to the Irish. He says Eddie is an idiot and needs to see a psychiatrist. Eddie tells him he *is* a psychiatrist and can he have a professional discount? The doctor gives him a prescription for an antibiotic and tells him next time he gets an infection from drinking beer upside down he should find another doctor. Eddie says, 'Thanks, Einstein.' "

As Tim told the story I could see the party: my brothers standing together, beers in their hands, heads thrown back, laughing; my aunts with their fox stoles wrapped around their necks and glasses of Old Fashioneds or Rob Roys on the table in front of them; two dozen little kids running around the house dodging between the clumps of adults scattered throughout the kitchen and dining room.

I hadn't seen Aunt Liz in two years, hadn't seen Eddie in four. When we moved to Rochester, Patti and I had left behind ten brothers, three sisters, nineteen aunts, fourteen uncles, and almost a hundred cousins. It had taken me a while, but I was finally starting to understand that the most important things in my life were back in Chicago. Patti had known this all along and had been waiting patiently for me to reach the same conclusion.

Back in January I had begun writing letters to orthopedic surgeons in Chicago. I called the chairman of orthopedics at Loyola where I went to medical school. I contacted several former Mayo residents who were now practicing in Chicago. Gradually we narrowed our choices down to two: a practice in Oak Park, where we both had been raised, or a practice a little farther west, in Hinsdale.

The Hinsdale practice was preferable in every way but one: the starting salary was terrible. If I accepted their offer I would be the lowest-paid resident to come out of Mayo that year. But what made the practice desirable was the opportunity it offered. For the first year I would still be an indentured servant, but after that I would be an equal partner, free to grow my practice as I saw fit. Ultimately we decided to ignore the lousy pay and accept the Hinsdale offer. We had been poor for so long that one more year of poverty didn't really matter to us.


We had a "new" car, an eight-year-old, wood-paneled Ford station wagon. We had purchased it two weeks earlier from Brian Quinn, a general surgery resident who was moving back to Ireland. The old Battleship, after surviving so many Minnesota winters, had died of spontaneous combustion in our garage one Friday morning. Mr. Jensen came over, looked at the charred mess where the engine used to be, slammed the hood, and "pronounced" it for us.

"It's over," he said. "This thing has burnt its last quart of oil. It's about time you got a new beater anyway. Hell, it's been almost two years now. You've got an image to keep up."

I thanked him and went in and called the junkyard.

"Jeez, Doc," Ernie Hausfeld said, "ain't heard from you in a while. Lemme guess, your new Mercedes's ashtray is full and you want to trade it in."

I told him no, I had another car for him.

"You're the damnedest doctor I've ever seen—driving all those junkers. Don't they pay you guys at Mayo?"

"Yeah, but I spend it all on whiskey and loose women."

Patti heard this and threw a stick of celery at me. "As if they'd have you," she said.

"Well," Ernie said, "it's the same deal. If you drive it in, you get thirty-five bucks. If we tow it in, you get twenty-five."

"Come on over," I said. "The old Battleship has set sail for the last time."

"It's called 'swallowing the anchor,' Doc."

"What?"

"Swallowing the anchor. It's an old Navy term. That's what we'd say when someone retired: they swallowed the anchor."

"Yeah, well swallow the anchor, gargle the bilge water, sleep wit' da fishes, whatever you want to call it, the old girl is dead."

Four hours later Jimmy pulled into our driveway. He had a big grin on his face.

"How's it going, Doc? Good t'see ya."

We shook hands.

"Ernie told me you're moving to Chicago. That's too bad. Hell, it won't be the same around here when you're gone." He hitched the winch to the front of the Battleship. "You're Ernie's best customer."

That's great. That will be my claim to fame: the resident who holds the all-time Mayo record for most cars towed to the junkyard. My parents will be so proud.

When Jimmy had the front of the Battleship off the ground and ready to go he turned to me. "See ya, Doc," he said. "Too bad we don't make house calls to Chicago. Guess you'll have to find a new junkyard." He waved a hand, hopped in the truck, and pulled out of the driveway, the old, rusted Battleship dangling from the crane.

Eileen watched him drive away. "Why is the man taking our car?" she asked.

"The car doesn't work anymore, honey," Patti told her.

"Can't the man fix it?"

"No, sweetie, the car is dead."

"Dead," she repeated. "Dead like Gramma?"

"Yes, like Gramma."

"Oh, goodie! Can we go to Chicago and have another party when they put the car in the ground?"

"No, Eileen, they don't put cars in the ground like they do people."

"Do they just put 'em in a box?"

"No, they don't put them in a box, either. They just leave them in a junkyard."

"Did they leave Gramma in—"

"No! Now go talk to your father."

Eileen looked inquiringly at me.

"Eileen," I said patiently, "you see, the car is not a person."

She nodded. "No, it's a sonna bitch."

"Eileen! That's a terrible thing to say," Patti said. "Where did you hear words like that?"

"That's what Daddy said yesterday when the car was making the smoke and bad noises."

Patti looked at me like *I* had just made smoke and bad noises. "Sometimes Daddy says things he shouldn't."

"Like when Notre Dame loses?"

God, the kid didn't forget anything.

"Yes. Sometimes Daddy says bad things then, too."

"We should wash his mouth out with soap."

"Well, maybe we should give Daddy another chance."

"Maybe Daddy should take this little squealer and drop her in a garbage can." I grabbed her and lifted her over my head. Eileen screamed and laughed as I held her poised over the garbage can. Mary Kate clapped and said Patrick was a stupid idiot and I should drop him in the garbage can, too. Patrick said Mary Kate was dog poop. Patti asked where we were going to get the money to buy another car. Jimmy came back and said I forgot to give him the title to the Battleship. Eileen saw the tow truck and said our dead car was back and maybe the man would bring our dead Gramma back, too. Mary Kate said Patrick put syrup in the toaster again. Jimmy took the title and said no one ever believes him when he tells them the things that go on at our house. Patti took the screwdriver out of Patrick's hand and pointed it at Jimmy. I told Jimmy he better take the title and leave before Patti's parole officer got there. Jimmy walked away, looking back over his shoulder every few steps. Patti told me it wasn't funny and people like Jimmy should mind their own business. Eileen told Mary Kate that Jimmy was a sonna bitch. Patti turned to me and said, "See what you started?"

It was a warm evening in late May, just past sunset. We had driven to Chicago for a dinner to meet my new partners. We had taken Maureen, who was only two weeks old, with us, but left her with Patti's sister for a few hours. We were cruising slowly down a two-lane road in Hinsdale, looking for the address on the invitation, when we saw the sign "3400" with an arrow pointing left. I turned down a dark, narrow road with huge, gnarled trees rising on either side, arching over the road and blotting out what little daylight was left. Ahead and to our right we could see lights.

"There," she pointed. "That must be it."

We came around the last curve, and there, on the crest of the hill before us, stood a brilliantly lit, stately, white-pillared home. I stopped the car and the two of us stared in disbelief. The home was splendid, magnificent, overwhelming. Neither of us had ever seen a home like that. It was like something out of the movies. We turned and looked at each other and then at this mansion in front of us.

"Are you sure this is the place?" Patti whispered, obviously afraid that Thurston Howell III was going to come out dressed in his silk smoking jacket and ascot. "Lovey," he would call over his shoulder, "some peasants are trespassing on our property." He would take a sip of his martini and, with a deprecating flick of the wrist, order us to remove ourselves, "and that thing you are driving," immediately.

"Look," I said, pointing at the small wooden sign next to the mailbox, "Thirty-four hundred. This is it."

Patti immediately started smoothing out her dress. She tilted the rearview mirror and checked her hair. "God, I look awful."

"Sure do," I said, trying not to laugh.

She slapped me on the shoulder and told me to shut up, that it wasn't funny, that there was no reason she should have to come to this stupid dinner anyway, that she never should have pulled her hair back that way in the first place, and that she could just kill Eileen for getting purple Magic Marker on her dress.

"You can't even see it," I said.

"You can too see it."

"Then perhaps Madame would like to slip into something more comfortable, *oui?*" I asked, raising my eyebrows and reaching for her.

"You stay away from me."

I patted her hand. "You look fine, hon. Stop worrying." I put the car back in gear and headed up the drive. "Now let's go meet everyone."

My new partners couldn't have been nicer. Their wives were equally gracious and welcoming. Within ten minutes Patti was laughing and chatting away with them like they had grown up together. We had a delightful dinner.

Pat took my arm as we were walking back to our car when the evening was over.

"They seem like nice people," she said.

"Yeah, they do. I guess we're pretty lucky to be joining a group like this."

When we reached our car, I turned back and stared at the house, feeling almost frightened by it.

"It's huge, isn't it?" I whispered.

"Yes."

The two of us stood there, uncertain how to confront the implications of what we were seeing.

"I don't want us to change," Patti said, laying her head against my shoulder.

I smiled, amazed at how accurately Patti could articulate my own feelings. We drove old, junky cars. We wore old, worn-out clothes. We never took vacations. We worked like dogs. And yet we didn't want to change. We already had everything we needed. We already had something so rare, so priceless, that we never wanted to lose it.

I slipped my arm around Patti and kissed her on the neck. "I don't want us to change, either," I said.

# CHAPTER FORTY

*June*

We drove back to Rochester the next morning. Dawn, the nursing student from next door, had stayed with the three older kids for the weekend. She was waiting at the door, suitcase in hand, when we came in. She looked glad to see us.

"They certainly are active little children," she said on her way out.

I had only three weeks left of my residency, but I still had to take call. As chief resident I could take call from home but I had to carry a beeper and I had to stay available. The following Friday night I had been asleep for two hours when the phone rang. It was Alan Harkins from the ER at St. Mary's.

"Sorry to wake you, Mike," he said, "but I need your help. The paramedics are bringing in a kid from Owatonna with a compound, comminuted tib-fib fracture. He's critical. They should be here in fifteen minutes."

I sat up, swung my legs over the side of the bed, and took a deep breath. "Okay, Alan," I said. "I'll be right there."

This was my last weekend on call. I had been hoping to make it through the night without getting called in; but I was so used to being called at night, so used to having my sleep interrupted, that I never gave it a thought. I pulled on a pair of pants and a sweatshirt and was at the hospital ten minutes later.

I had just changed into my scrubs when the ER doors crashed open and the paramedics powered through. I trotted alongside them as they wheeled the patient to Trauma One.

"Fourteen-year-old kid, run over by a tractor," the paramedic said. "He was conscious when we got there, BP a hundred over sixty. But his right leg's a mess—open fracture, dirt everywhere."

A fourteen-year-old kid on a tractor at midnight? God, I thought, these farm kids work hard.

"What's his name?" I asked.

"Johannson. Kenny Johannson."

"Hang in there, Kenny," I whispered to the unconscious boy.

I lifted the sheet covering the lower half of his body, and immediately the thick, fetid stink of manure mushroomed up at me. The leg was twisted obscenely to the side. The jagged end of the tibia stuck through a rent in his dirty blue jeans. A spreading pool of blood soaked the sheet underneath him.

As we lifted the boy onto the table in Trauma One, his eyes flickered open. He began to whimper softly as he searched for someone he knew. I put my hand on the side of his head and rubbed his hair gently. "Kenny, you're in the emergency room at St. Mary's," I told him. "Your mom and dad are here, too. They're in the other room."

He rolled his head and moaned. "My leg. Oh, God, my leg! It hurts so bad."

"I know it does, Kenny, and we are going to help you."

"BP seventy-eight over forty," a nurse called out. "Pulse one-sixty."

I probed Kenny's wound. Under the severed end of the peroneus longus there was a bloody chunk of manure wedged against the bone. I picked it up with a forceps and dropped it on the floor. When I found what was left of the anterior tibial artery I clipped it with a hemostat. His bleeding, except for a slow ooze, ceased.

In the next several minutes we did a cut-down, put in a subclavian line, and pumped him full of blood and fluid. Within half an hour we had his pressure up to one-ten over sixty. I told the charge nurse to get an OR ready. As she picked up the phone, she said when I got a chance the parents wanted to talk to me.

Mr. and Mrs. Johannson were huddled together on a couch in the far corner of the waiting room. They sprang to their feet as I entered the waiting room. Mrs. Johannson wrapped both hands around her husband's left arm and leaned against him. She kept staring at the bloodstains on my pants.

I introduced myself and then told them that although Kenny had lost a lot of blood, his vital signs had improved and he seemed stable. "We are just about to take him to the operating room," I said.

Before I could say more, the door to the waiting room burst open and a young man rushed in. "Dad," he said, "I found it."

"This is my son, Eric," Mr. Johannson said. "He went back to the farm to look for the missing piece of Kenny's leg."

Eric reached into the pocket of his jacket. He handed me a clean white handkerchief in which he had wrapped a dirty, three-inch section of tibia. I doubted we could use it, but I wanted the boy to feel he had done something worthwhile. "Thanks Eric," I said. "This could be a big help."

"Will you be able to save Kenny's leg?" Mr. Johannson asked.

At that moment I was more worried about saving Kenny's life. The boy was in shock and had almost bled to death. I longed to reassure his parents, but I had learned not to make promises. "Mr. Johannson," I said, "we're going to do everything we can."

"Please, Doc. Please."

I nodded, shook his hand, squeezed Mrs. Johannson's shoulder, and sprinted up to the OR.


They had taken Kenny to OR Ten, the largest of the operating rooms. In contrast to the ER where everyone had been barking orders, shouting for equipment, and rushing back and forth, the operating room was quiet, almost hushed. Voices were muffled. There was a greater sense of control here. We were surgeons. This was our turf.

Against the far wall the laminar-flow machine hummed faintly. The cardiac monitor issued its staccato, reassuring beeps. Two anesthesiologists were wedged shoulder to shoulder at the head of the table. They had just finished the intubation. The scrub nurse stood at the back table carefully arranging her instruments. Two circulating nurses shuttled back and forth with instrument trays from the sterilizer. In the corner, a radiology tech waited patiently next to her portable X-ray machine.

I handed the piece of tibia to the circulating nurse and asked her to sterilize it. Then I scrubbed my hands and joined the five other residents from various surgical specialties who were clustered around the shattered leg. The extent of the boy's injuries was now apparent. Large sections of muscle, skin, and bone were missing. Parts of nerves and arteries had been torn away. Dirt, manure, and fertilizer contaminated everything.

First one, then another of the residents poked at the wound, winced or shook his head, then stepped back. No one was sure what to do. Should we try to save this leg, or should we amputate it?

They all looked at me. I was the chief resident in Orthopedic Surgery. I was the one who had to decide.

I stood in the center of the operating room with the bright lights trained on the bloody mess that was Kenny's leg. I tried to put everything else out of my mind. It didn't matter how much sleep I got last night. It didn't matter what else I had planned for the rest of the day. This poor kid, barely alive, was lying unconscious on an operating table with some stranger about to decide whether to cut off his leg.

I hemmed and hawed for a few minutes. The natural impulse, of course, is to save the leg. If there is a chance in a million, take it. The kid was only fourteen years old. What did we have to lose by trying? If it didn't work we could always amputate the leg later. Didn't we owe him at least that much?

I wasn't sure. Kenny's leg was so badly damaged that an attempt to save his leg could cost him his life.

But what about Kenny? What would *he* want? If we woke him up and said, "Kenny, your leg is severely injured. Should we cut it off or try to save it?" Does anyone think he would say, "Cut it off"?

For Christ's sake, he was only fourteen years old.

The room was quiet save for the sigh of the ventilator and the steady beep of the cardiac monitor. From behind the drape at the head of the table, the anesthesiologists looked at me questioningly. The other residents stood silent, some looking at the ground, some staring at the gaping wound in front of us. No one moved. No one spoke. They all waited.

On the surgical field in front of me was a leg. That's all that could be seen. The draping was deliberately arranged to exclude everything else. Everything else was superfluous. In hiding the rest of the body, the rest of reality, we were trying to convince ourselves, as surgeons always do, that we had defined and isolated the problem to the mangled hunk of skin and bone on the sterile, blue surgical sheet in front of us. It was so much cleaner, so much easier, that way.

But what of life's unseen tendrils that spread slowly from this leg, extending under the drapes, out of the room, and into the unpredictable world we tried so tenaciously to exclude? What of Kenny's basketball games, and high school dances? What of the walks in the woods, and the sensuous intermingling of legs on his first night of sex? Did we really think by hanging sterile blue sheets in a room on the second floor of a hospital we were no longer required to think of those things, too?

This was not some abstract problem of surgical technique or diagnosis. This was not even a dispassionate analysis of the viability of muscle tissue or the regenerative ability of nerves. This was deciding whether to amputate a kid's leg. This required an understanding that an amputation means more than just severing bone, muscle, and tendon. This required an understanding of what a scalpel can and can't do.

I knew there was an easy out. I could say it was the kid's decision, not mine. I could step back, hold up my hands, and say, "Don't blame me. I just did what Kenny wanted."

Or was it?

No, I realized, that's *not* what Kenny, or his parents, wanted. What they wanted was a compassionate, highly trained surgeon who would do what he thought was in the best interest of this little boy. And I knew what was in the best interest of this little boy. I knew damn well. I just didn't want to do it.

Go ahead, I told myself. Be the hero. Fix the kid's leg. You'll be four hundred miles away six months from now when Kenny and his family realize they should have had an amputation. Someone else will have to do the dirty work then. But the family will always remember you as the hero, the surgeon who saved Kenny's leg.

I looked at the mutilated pile of skin and bone that up until two hours ago had been a miracle of functioning flesh. Now it was only a mass of dark meat lying on a blue surgical sheet slowly oozing its life away.

I picked up a scalpel and began the amputation.

It was 4:30 A.M. by the time we wheeled Kenny into the recovery room. His vitals were stable. It looked as though he would make it. His parents, his brother, and some aunts and uncles stood up when I came into the waiting room. I told them Kenny had made it through surgery and although he was still in critical condition we thought he would pull through.

"What about his leg?" the father asked.

I looked at them, struggling to find words. My hesitation confirmed their worst fears. "I'm afraid the injuries to Kenny's leg were just too severe," I began. "There was no way . . ." When I told them I had to amputate the leg, Kenny's mother's hand flew to her mouth. His father's shoulders sagged and he hung his head.

"But," I said, "there is an excellent chance that he will walk quite normally with a prosthesis." I said a few more things about Kenny needing a lot of support during the next few weeks, but they didn't seem to hear much after the part about the amputation. I could see the disappointment, the accusation in their eyes. Why hadn't I saved Kenny's leg? Why had I failed them?

When I finished talking to the family I went back to the doctors' locker room. It was 4:50. I considered lying down on the couch until rounds at 7:30, but decided instead to go home. The thought of two hours in my own bed was too good to pass up. I was going to leave my scrubs on, but saw there was blood spattered all over my pants and shoes, so I changed and then headed home.

A light, sleety rain was falling as I walked through the empty parking lot to my car. I stood for a moment, key in the door, lifting my face and letting the soft rain wash over me. Swirls of sleet drifted past the light above me. It felt good just to be out there. It felt good to rediscover that life isn't all pain and suffering. I was glad I decided to go home, and to leave all those other things behind—at least for a while.

I closed my eyes, enfolded in the soothing caress of the rain. A few seconds later I swayed against the side of the car. My eyes snapped open. Home, I thought. I need to go home.

I turned and looked back at the brilliantly lit emergency room entrance. An ambulance was parked there, its doors open. It was empty, but an air of tension lingered in the air. A seat belt dangled from the driver's side. From the radio receiver in the front seat I could hear garbled voices, urgent transmissions about other emergencies in other places. In the back of the ambulance I could see a blood pressure cuff swinging back and forth from a silver hook on the wall. The floor was littered with empty syringes and vials, a plastic airway, and ten or twenty bloody 4×4s.

On another night I would have been inside as the patient was wheeled in. I could see the ERSS chief barking orders, the junior resident wiping back the hair from his forehead as he tried to get an IV started. Someone else was prepping the chest for the subclavian line. Techs were scurrying back and forth with blood tests and X-rays.

Not tonight, I thought. Tonight it's their show, not mine. I'm going home.

I opened the car door, dropped into the driver's seat, and headed west on Second St. I knew the heater would never warm up in the five minutes it took to drive home so I scrunched down in the front seat, shivering slightly. At least the wipers were working. In the rearview mirror a faint gray was spreading across the dark sky as night dripped slowly into day.

What a life, I thought. What a crazy life. Going home at five o'clock in the morning excited because I have a chance to sleep in my own bed for two hours.

As the car splashed on I began thinking how much my life had changed in the last few years. I thought about all the guys I had grown up with. I still got together with them every Christmas when I was home. They were the same old guys. They partied and laughed. They shot pool at O'Dea's, went to Sox games, played sixteen-inch softball, and closed Callahan's on Saturday night. Yes, they, too, were getting married, finding jobs, starting families; and yes, they, too, put in some long hours. But at least their lives had some balance. At least they didn't have to worry that every mistake they made would kill or cripple someone.

I remembered all the times, so very long ago it seemed, when I was one of those guys—single, roaming the bars on the West Side, shooting pool and singing Irish songs, closing one pub and going to another until the last bartender at the last bar served us the very last beer. ("Time now! Time, gents! For the love o' Jaysus, it's half three. Have yez no homes to go to? I mean it, lads. This is the last one. Get ye home.") God, it seemed like another life, another person. Was that really me?

I liked the person I was ten years ago. But I wasn't sure I liked this new person, this surgeon, I had become. Who was he? I had never gotten to know him. I hadn't the time. Time was a tool I used to accomplish other, bigger things. I had learned to manage my time so efficiently, to be so perfectly pragmatic and utilitarian. Introspection was an irrelevance, and I had no time for irrelevance.

Perhaps because it was so late and I was silly from lack of sleep, I began to wonder what it would be like to meet my old self. I was approaching the point where Second St. leaves the city and becomes a country road. Under the last streetlight I imagined I saw someone. It was myself, my *younger* self, standing in the rain, his Notre Dame letter jacket hunched up around his neck. His thumb was out, and he was trying to hitch a ride. I stopped to pick him up. I knew him and he knew me. He got in the backseat, slammed the door, and shook the rain from his wet hair.

"Thanks," he said, trying not to be too obvious, as he looked me over. He seemed rather deferential at first, almost as if he were in awe of me— perhaps because it was hard for him to imagine himself being so different and yet so much the same. He felt at a disadvantage. I knew everything about him but he knew nothing about me. He stared at me, wondering how such a profound change could come about. He couldn't tell yet if he was pleased with this change or not. He asked me what I did.

"I'm a doctor."

He looked at me in amazement. He thought I was kidding. The possibility of becoming a doctor had never entered his mind. He leaned forward and put his hand on the front seat. I could smell the beer on his breath.

"Really. A doctor, huh?"

"Yeah."

"What kind of doctor?"

"An orthopedic surgeon." I only say "orthopedic surgeon" when I'm trying to impress someone. Otherwise I just call myself an orthopod.

"Orthopedic," he said. "That's a bone doctor, right?"

"Yeah. Bones and joints."

"Jeez." He was quiet for a minute, then asked, "So, are you married?"

"Yeah."

"You are?" He seemed even more surprised and delighted. He wanted to know everything about Patti—what she looked like, how we met, where she was from. When I told him we had four kids he stared at me in amazement.

"Honest to God," he whispered almost to himself. "A wife and four kids." He sat there, looking out the window into the rain, a faint smile on his face.

We were quiet then, each of us looking from a different perspective at the direction my life had taken. As we splashed on through the night I noticed him squirming around in the backseat. I thought I knew what might be the matter.

"I see a rural men's room up ahead," I said, pointing to a large bush on the side of the road. "Looks like I'd better pull over."

The car grated to a stop on the shoulder, next to the bush. He pushed the door open, then leaned forward and held out his hand. As we shook hands he thanked me for the ride and said, "You take care of Patti and those kids, okay?"

I laughed. "You don't even know Patti," I said.

He stepped out of the car, then put his hand on the door and leaned back in. "You heard what I said. I don't care about all your doctor shit. That stuff's fine, but you take care of Patti first."

He eyed me steadily. I knew that look. And suddenly I knew I was the one being judged.

"Don't worry," I said. "I will."

"Good."

He was still looking at me, but was shifting his weight from foot to foot.

"Go on," I said, pointing to the bush, "get out of here before you have an accident."

He stared at me for a few seconds, as if he wanted to remember all this, as if he were afraid that if he didn't hold on to this moment it would turn out to be a dream. Finally, he slammed the door, raised his hand in farewell, and began to trot away. As he rounded the corner of the bush, I could hear him break into a familiar song: *"For freedom comes from God's right hand, and needs a goodly train—"*

*"And righteous men must make our land a nation once again,"* I sang with him.

I pulled away, glad for the vote of confidence; glad at least someone thought I had turned out all right.

# CHAPTER FORTY-ONE

*June*

The annual Orthopedic Residents' Farewell Dinner was held in the Banquet Room of the Holiday Inn. There was a cocktail hour (that stretched into two), a steak and baked potato dinner, and lots of speeches by the junior residents about what great guys the departing residents were. We lifted our glasses and said, "Damn right." The juniors even put on a slide show, a take-off on *The Odyssey* complete with a Cyclops who bore a striking resemblance to BJ Burke, and the Sirens whose faces had been changed to those of the ortho nurses.

The bar stayed open before, during, and after dinner. Everyone kept buying us beers, and slapping us on the back, and saying how much they were going to miss us. Jack Manning came back from the bathroom with a top hat he got from a guy at a wedding. Bill Chapin left and came back wearing a tiara he got from a girl at the state baton convention. "It goes with my tie, don't you think?" he asked Patti.

Patti said it looked very nice, but she hoped he wasn't driving home. "In fact," she said, "I hope *none* of you are."

When the night was over I solemnly shook hands with Jack and Frank and Bill. Then I told them all to shut up. I had something important to say. I was swaying a little as I began. I said I would never forget all the times they held my beeper while I was moonlighting. "Patti and I couldn't have made it without you," I said. "You guys are like brothers to me."

Frank said thanks, but he didn't need any Irish Catholic brothers with twenty kids.

Linda gave Frank a slap on the shoulder and said, "Mike and Patti don't need any wisecracks from you." Alice Chapin gave me a big kiss and told me to "take good care of Patti or I'll kill you." Sue Manning said she loved me, but there already were enough Irish Catholic babies in Chicago and would I please leave Patti alone?

"Yeah," Jack said. "Like Groucho Marx used to say: 'I like my cigar, but I take it out of my mouth once in a while.' "

Sue told him he was crude and should keep his mouth shut.

Then Jack started blubbering that we were the greatest bunch of guys in the world, and would we sing "The Ballad of the Green Berets" with him? We did, even though no one knew the words except Jack.

Frank, who had a beautiful voice, sang some sad cowboy song where everyone gets killed except the horse. When he finished he said he would have a place for us back on his ranch anytime we wanted to visit. "Any one of you," he repeated, "anytime. Even you and your twenty kids, Collins," he said, putting his arm around me. Then he walked over to Patti, kissed her, and said she should come—without me.

Since everyone was singing, I gave them "A Nation Once Again" Jack said it was a stupid song and what was the point since Irishmen were always going to fight no matter what and it was better they fought each other and left the rest of the world alone.

Bill adjusted his tiara and said we were a bunch of bums, and he wouldn't let a single one of us operate on his dog. Then he bought another round.


We were going our separate ways. Bill was joining a large, multispecialty group in Missouri. Frank was headed back to Wyoming to a three-man practice near Jackson Hole. Jack Manning had been asked to stay on staff at Mayo.

"They took Manning, but I'm really the one they wanted," Bill said.

By now our wives had managed to get us as far as the parking lot. They stood there, arms folded, waiting. "Yeah, the big shots at the Clinic were on the phone to me every damn day for a month," Bill went on. "But I know my old buddy, Jack, can't find a job. So I go to BJ Burke. 'BJ,' I say, 'we need to talk. Me and you. *Mano y mano.* It's about Jack Manning. He can't find a job. No one will hire the dumb son of a bitch. We gotta do something, BJ. As a personal favor to me do you think you could find a spot for him here at Mayo?'

"Well, old BJ hands me a big, honking Cuban cigar. 'Bill,' he says, holding a match to my stogie, 'never mind this Manning character. You're the brightest star in the orthopedic constellation. What will it take to get you to stay on staff here?'

"I put my arm around him. 'BJ,' I say, 'you got a nice place here. Very nice. I'd love to help you out, but I'm a ramblin', gamblin', Vegas kinda guy, and I gotta be movin' on. I would take it very kindly if you gave Manning a job, though. He could see all the infected, hypochondriac, workman's comp cases.'

"BJ shakes his head sadly. 'Manning!' he says. I can see the disappointment in his eyes. Finally he straightens up, sighs and says, 'All right, Bill. I'll do this for you—but you owe me, big time.'"

"Chapin," Jack said, "what did you do before they invented bullshit?"

The farewell dinner was over, but no one wanted to say good-bye. We stood silently under the soft glow of a light in the parking lot, four guys trying to make time stand still. We didn't want this night, this chapter in our lives, to end. We stared at the ground or looked off into the dark night, unable to look at one another. Gathered at the exit of the Holiday Inn, our wives waited patiently, watching us with amusement and exasperation—but they didn't want this night to end, either. Like us, they knew that when we said good night and piled into our cars we would be calling an end to a lot of things.

We stood there feeling like the patient who thinks he has cancer but refuses to let his doctor do a biopsy, reasoning that he can't have cancer unless the biopsy proves it's cancer, so if he refuses to allow the biopsy he won't have cancer. If we didn't say good night, if we just kept standing there in the parking lot, we could stay friends and residents forever. We, who had been grumbling for four years about ortho dogs and lousy pay and scut work and ignominy, now couldn't bear to see it all come to an end.

Finally, our wives came over.

"Come on, Jack," Sue said softly, "we should go."

Jack nodded but said nothing. He stood with his head bowed, gently kicking at an invisible spot on the asphalt.

Patti laid her hand on my shoulder. "Mike," she said, her eyes gently pleading, "it's quarter to three."

I looked at her and smiled. "You sound like one of the old bartenders at O'Dea's," I said. "Next you'll be asking, 'Have yez no homes to go to?'"

I let out a long, slow breath and then turned to Frank Wales. "Well, cowboy, I guess it's time to saddle up and get out of Dodge."

Frank nodded. "Four years," he said slowly. "Well, it's sure been a pleasure, Mike, a gol dern pleasure."

I clapped Bill Chapin on the back. "Take care of that pudendal nerve, okay?"

Bill cracked a smile and told me to screw off.

It was time, and we knew it. I set my bottle of Grain Belt on the hood of the car next to me and shook hands one last time with Bill and Frank and Jack. I kissed and hugged Alice and Linda and Sue.

Then Patti took me home.

# CHAPTER FORTY-TWO

*The end of June*

It was my last day as chief resident. There was no graduation ceremony, no cap and gown, no pomp and circumstance. There wasn't even a diploma. We were just supposed to pack our things and leave. I met a couple residents in the hall. They were too busy to stop and talk but they clapped me on the back and wished me well. I went up to the residents' lounge to clean out my locker and mailbox. Next to the mailboxes, in an old, overstuffed armchair, a resident in a rumpled blue sport coat was sound asleep, his head lolled to the right, his mouth slightly open.

I had handed my beeper to the operator at St. Mary's earlier that afternoon, and for the first time in four years, was not given another to take its place. The educational odyssey that had begun in high school seventeen years before was over. The most prestigious medical center in the world had signed off on me, had told the world I was ready.

I didn't feel ready. Oh, sure, I was a god to the junior residents—just as the graduating chiefs had been gods to me when I was a junior resident. But I still had so much to learn. When was I going to feel the equal of Cuv or Tom Hale or Antonio Romero?

Patti and I were sitting next to each other on the swing set in the backyard, not saying much. We had just come from the closing. Tomorrow night another family would be sleeping in our house.

"The raspberries should be ready to pick in another week," I said, nodding at the patch in the corner of the yard.

"We won't be here in another week."

I could tell without looking she was crying. She was digging around in her pockets for a Kleenex. I don't know why. She never carried one. I passed her my handkerchief.

She wiped her eyes and then said, "Can I have a hug?"

We each stepped off our swing and I put my arms around her.

"This is so nice," she said, her head on my chest.

This is how I want to leave the world, I thought. I don't care if I'm rich or famous; just let me die with my arms around Patti.

We were silent for a long time. I knew what was on her mind, though. "I hate to leave, hon," I said. "Don't you?"

"Yes," she said. "I cried because we had to come here, and now I'm crying because we have to leave."

She looked at me and smiled. That was Patti, putting on the brave face and doing what needed to be done. I never told her how it broke my heart to see her with that sad smile. I guess no one ever told her that smiles and tears don't go together.

"Well," I said, kissing her on the forehead, "I guess I'd better get going. Are you sure you're going to be all right?"

"Yes," Patti said, "we'll be fine."

It was Friday night. The movers were coming the next morning. But the movers wanted money; and as usual, we had no money. The movers said if we didn't have a certified check waiting for them on Monday morning when they got to Chicago they would not unload the truck.

We had no money, but we had a plan. Patti would supervise the move, and then drive to Chicago in the station wagon with the kids. Meanwhile, I would borrow a car, drive to Mankato, and do a marathon moonlighting session: 7:00 P.M. Friday night until 5:00 A.M. Monday morning. When I finished, I would drive back to Rochester, drop off the car, fly to Chicago, go to our new bank, deposit my moonlighting check, get a cashier's check, and then meet the movers at our new home.

And that is just how it happened. Patti supervised the loading of the furniture the next day. Then Mrs. Flaherty, whose daughter, Mary, had been our babysitter ever since we moved to Rochester, came over and sprinkled the car, Patti, and each of the kids with holy water, praying for a safe trip.

They arrived safe and sound at Patti's parents' house at eight o'clock that night, after four bathroom stops, three dirty diapers, and one episode of vomit—Patrick never liked the backseat.

I, meanwhile, was moonlighting in Mankato. At 3:30 Saturday morning an ambulance brought in a guy with a cervical spine fracture. I stabilized him, then called Mayo to arrange a transfer. Steve DeBurke was the ortho resident on call. He had just finished Basic Science and was a senior resident now.

"Is this *the* Dr. Collins, formerly of the Mayo Clinic?" Steve asked.

*Formerly.* It felt strange to hear him say it like that. But he was right. I was no longer one of them. A new group of residents, fresh from medical school, would start that morning. All my friends, all my fellow residents, were gone. Bill, Frank, Jack, and all the others had packed up and moved on. Their days as residents were over. But I was still there, still working. I was the last of us, the last resident.

"You know, I just thought of something," I said. "I am no longer employed by the Mayo Clinic. I don't start my new job 'til next week. I've sold my home and don't close on the new one 'til Monday. So, right now I'm thirty-four years old. I'm married. I've got four kids, and I have no job, no home, and no money."

Steve yawned loudly. "Did you call me at three o'clock in the morning to tell me this sob story?"

"No, I didn't. I've got a guy with a C-5 burst fracture. He's neurologically intact, but the fracture is unstable."

"No problem. Just ship him over."

When Connie Fritz came on duty on Sunday night she said, "You know this is sick, don't you?" Connie had been working the night shift at St. Joe's for twenty-seven years. She and I had become very close over the past four years. "I worked with you Friday night," she said, "then I went home and slept, did some shopping and visited the grandkids. I worked with you Saturday night, then I went home and slept, went to church, and had dinner at my sister's. Now I come back on Sunday night and you're still here. You look like shit, you know. What the hell is wrong with you to work like this?"

I told Connie it wasn't so bad. I had slept a little here and there.

"Slept a little my ass. Have fun dying when you're forty," she said.

"If I do, will you come to Chicago and raise my kids?" I asked.

"I'll come to Chicago and piss on your grave."


By Monday morning at five I had been working fifty-eight straight hours. I had managed a few hours of sleep, but was coasting in on fumes, stubble-chinned, bleary-eyed, and working by instinct. I was neither awake nor asleep, neither alive nor dead—a condition not unlike that in which I had spent much of the past four years. I shuffled dumbly from one task to the next: peering in infected ears, palpating painful bellies, auscultating ischemic hearts, repairing jagged lacerations.

I liked repairing lacerations the best. I could turn off my brain, and function at some simian, subcortical level, frowning in concentration as I slowly, deliberately placed each stitch, the delicate twist of the wrist bringing the needle into and out of the edges of the laceration. There was a numbing rhythm to the ratcheting click of the needle-holder, the snip of the scissors, the silent daub of the gauze. There was something comfortingly bourgeois and reaffirming in suturing lacerations: mindless, repetitive steps proceeding to a defined goal; the edges of the laceration slowly coming together, stitch by stitch.

When I finished the repair, I wiped away the last bit of blood, carefully dressed the wound, then stood up. I was suddenly lost, out of focus. What now?

With nothing immediately demanding my attention, I found myself incapable of attending to anything at all. I desperately wanted to be done, to close my eyes, to rest, and yet I was painfully aware that I actually *liked* this, and in thirty minutes it would be gone forever.

When the last drunk was stitched, the last chest pain admitted, the last antibiotic prescribed, I tossed the prescription pad on the counter, threw my lab coat in the laundry basket, and kissed the nurses good-bye. I was swallowing the anchor.

Connie handed me a cup of coffee and said, "Now get out of here, you big lunk." Then she and the other nurses gathered in the doorway and waved to me as I drove out of the parking lot. "Drive carefully, Doctor." "Take care of those kids." "Come back and see us sometime."

I rolled down the windows, unbuttoned my shirt, turned up the radio, and headed east, into the rising sun, going back to Rochester one last time. In a dreamlike, sleep-deprived state I drifted along, flooded with memories. Eagle Lake, Smith's Mill, Janesville, there wasn't a town along the way that didn't have someone I had stitched up or casted or repaired or resuscitated. I felt a fondness for them all, and a sense of gratitude that I had been able to help them. It had been a lot of work. At times it felt like I was killing myself. And yet the only thing I could recall at that moment was how much fun it had been, and how wonderful it was to do this for a living.

I managed, barely, to stay awake on the ride back to Rochester, but almost missed the flight.

"You'd better hurry," the lady at check-in told me. "The plane's about to depart."

I tried to sprint down the gangway, but my legs wouldn't do what I told them. The flight attendant was starting to close the door to the plane as I stumbled up to her. She looked at me curiously, checked my ticket, and motioned me in. I mumbled my thanks, staggered down the aisle, dropped into my seat, and finally closed my eyes.

*Urrr.*

There was a noise. A noise from far away.

*Urrr.*

It was a voice.

"Sir," the voice was saying.

I opened my eyes. The voice was coming from a face. Why was there a face in front of me?

"Sir, the plane has landed. You have to get off now."

Plane? Landed?

"Sir, are you okay?"

"Okay," I said.

"We're in Chicago. You have to get off now."

"Have to get off now." I got to my feet and stumbled into the aisle. The plane was empty.

"Sir, is that your bag?"

"My bag? Yes, my bag. Thank you."

My brother Tim was waiting for me. I had no luggage. Tim took me to the bank, where I got the cashier's check. Then he dropped me off at our new home. Patti and the kids were already there.

Patti was looking at me funny.

"What?" I said.

"I was trying to remember why I married you."

I rubbed a hand over my chin. "It was for my dashing good looks, my savoir faire, my—"

"Do you have the check?"

"Check? What check?"

"Don't make me hurt you."

It was nine o'clock. The movers got out of the truck. They stretched, yawned, and sauntered over. Patti was on a first-name basis with all of them. They, of course, loved her. She had laughed with them, gossiped about the Twins and the White Sox, and had given them cookies, pop, and beer when they loaded the truck in Rochester. They, in turn, played with the kids, learned their names, and heard the story of the strange husband who was going to work three days and three nights in a row to pay for the move.

"So you made it, huh, Doc?" the mover said as he folded the cashier's check and put it in his shirt pocket.

"Yeah, I made it."

"Did you ever sleep?"

"Some."

"Well, here's your receipt," he said, handing me a sheet of paper. "We're going to need you to sign a few things when we're done."

"I might not be here."

"Huh? Where else you gonna be?"

"Asleep."

"Oh, yeah," he said with a laugh. "Say, wait 'til you see this." He lifted a heavy bar and swung open the back door of the moving van. The first thing I saw was our bed. "Patti made sure it was the last thing we loaded on the truck. She said you might be needing it."

Just then Patrick ran up and slapped the mover a high five. "Hiya, Ollie!" he said.

"Hi, short legs. You gonna help us move this stuff?"

"Evewything," he said, throwing his arms in the air.

In ten minutes we had the bed assembled in our room. Patti, who thought of everything, even had a set of sheets and a blanket for it.

"That sure is some woman you're married to," the mover said to me.

"Patti? She's the best."

I sagged down on the bed, curled my arm under the pillow, and closed my eyes. As my last bit of consciousness faded, I realized how lucky I was; and I knew that everything I had to endure over the last four years—the long hours, the lousy pay, the studying, the moonlighting, the nights on call—was worth it. Every bit of everything I had to endure was worth it.

The mover picked up the last of his tools and switched off the light. I was asleep before he closed the door.

# AUTHOR'S NOTE

It is the peculiar lot of the memoirist to respect truth without shackling himself to literality. This is especially so in the medical field, where the interests of the patient must always be respected. Out of concern for the privacy of both my colleagues and my patients I have changed the names and descriptions of all characters in this book, with the exception of my family members and Mark Coventry. Dr. Coventry died a few years ago. I feel privileged to have known and worked with him, and I thought my portrayal of him was so laudatory that he wouldn't mind that I used his real name.

I also hope my affection and respect for the Mayo Clinic and the wonderful, dedicated orthopedic surgeons who taught me, came through. Mayo is, indeed, the best medical center in the world. It was my privilege to train there.

Some thanks are in order. First of all to my wife, Patti, and all the kids: Eileen, Mary Kate, Paudh, Maureen, Sheila, Kevin, Matt, Nora, Brian, Ann, Katie, and Colleen. They listened to or read, laughed or cried with me through the several years it took to write this book. Thank you all for your help and encouragement. To the little ones I will say again: just because you hear or read bad words doesn't mean you have to use them.

In the professional arena special thanks go to my agent, Meg Ruley, who has been everything an author could desire.

And one last thing. I wouldn't want to close without a final note to Bill Chapin, Frank Wales, and Jack Manning. You know who you are, and I'll say it again: Patti and I couldn't have made it without you guys. Thanks.